The Philosophy of Dieting

Lose weight and look great with the help of philosophers from Plato to Camus

Peter Hayes

Published by

Gilbert Knowle Publishers
6 Valeside
Durham DH1 4RF

© Peter Hayes 2012

ISBN: 978-0-9558815-7-2

Contents

To Toshie

Introduction

All around there are people trying to make you feel *bad* for being overweight. They claim that they are anxious about your health, about heart disease, diabetes, and so on, and they ask you accusingly what *you* are going to do to help solve the international obesity crisis. Sometimes diet books are not much better, particularly the ones that scare their readers by describing all the health problems that overweight people can have. But I am not sure that anyone *really* cares. All those po-faced warnings over the dangers of being fat, all the hand wringing, they are not truly motivated by a altruistic concern about your health. No. When someone makes you feel bad about your weight, the real reason why they do it is simple: making you feel bad makes *them* feel good.

So I am not going to spend my time telling you about how awful it is to be overweight. I want you to lose weight because you love the idea of being slim, not because you are afraid to be fat. And I want to get a couple things absolutely straight right at the start. First, *there is nothing wrong with being overweight.* Second, this book has been written to help you lose weight, but *not to make you feel bad about your weight.* If you are overweight and are happy about that, then good for you! You have certainly got your priorities right because there are plenty of things out there that are far more important than what you happen to weigh.

It is true that the overweight have a shorter life expectancy. But we all have to die sometime, and almost every philosopher since Socrates gives the same message: It is not how *long* you live that is important, it is how *well* you live. If you are fat and happy, then that is a pretty good sign that you are living well; you're charting your own course and not spending your whole time trying to follow the herd. In the words of the ancient Himalayan proverb 'Better to live for one day as a tiger than for a thousand years as a sheep.' And this proverb is every bit as valid if the 'tiger' is a roly-poly one.

If there's nothing wrong with being an overweight tiger then why write a whole book about how philosophers can help you to diet? Why lose weight at all? The answer is that while there is nothing wrong with being overweight, there *is* something wrong with being unhappy, so this is a book for people who are overweight and unhappy about it. If that describes you then cheer up! This book is all you need. Follow its instructions and I guarantee you will lose weight.* And not only that, you will *enjoy* losing weight. Dieting does not have to be a grind. It can be fun. And philosophers, yes, *philosophers,* are the people who will make dieting fun for you!

Meet the Philosophers

Our philosophers are in two main groups, first there are the nice ones and second the Four Germans. Let's go to the nice philosophers first.

In Chapter One we meet Henri Bergson, a French philosopher of the early twentieth century. A lot of people look down their nose at him now because he criticised Darwin and Einstein. Whether he was right or wrong to challenge these scientists (I think he was right), Bergson was certainly brave in the face of evil. When France surrendered to the

---

* It must be admitted that, like most guarantees, this guarantee is worthless, because if you say. 'Hey! I have not lost any weight,' then I will just say: 'Well that just proves you didn't follow the instructions properly!'

Nazis, he insisted on registering himself as a Jew, even though he did not have to. But before he could be murdered he died of a cold at the age of 81. Bergson's books are about free will, time, society, simultaneity, memory, life, and ... laughter! So he gives us the laughter diet. This chapter comes first because it provides a key underlying principle that informs all our diets: *philosophical dieting is lighted hearted.* This means that if you can laugh about a diet *this will help that diet to work.*

In Chapter Two we go back to classical Athens to meet Plato, probably the world's greatest philosopher, and Socrates, who never wrote anything down himself but whom we learn about through Plato. This is where the philosophy of dieting really gets going, because Plato gives an amazingly powerful explanation for why we are overweight. Philosophers after Plato all know this, and many of their ideas about how to diet build on his insights.

Then we jump forward two thousand years to consider how Thomas Hobbes and René Descartes can help us to formulate a diet contract (Chapter Three). Hobbes was a seventeenth century 'social contract' thinker who said that all he wanted to do was to warn people to obey the law. This project sounds innocent, but the way Hobbes argued his case was so subversive that he frightened kings and infuriated bishops. When things got too hot for him, Hobbes always managed to escape, though they did burn a few of his books. Descartes explores the mind-body problem, and has some very helpful advice about how to make our body weigh less by expanding the power of our minds.

In Chapter Four we turn to John Locke who provided the philosophical foundations of the American Constitution. By exploring Locke's work, we discover that as well as setting out the principles on which the United States is governed, he also propounded a slightly indelicate but highly effective method of dieting, and that we can follow this diet with the help of a bucket.

After looking at the diets proposed by these (relatively) nice philosophers we move on to the Four Germans, starting with Karl Marx (Chapter Five). Despite his cuddly teddy bear good looks, Marx is also one of the most bloodthirsty of the great philosophers and his revolutionary diet is slightly disturbing. We follow this in Chapter Six with Georg Wilhelm Friedrich Hegel, whose books are about the clash of opposites, including the clash between being fat and being thin. In Chapter Seven we consider Arthur Schopenhauer who is famous (or infamous) as a misogynist or women-hater. Beneath this surface hostility, Schopenhauer is surprisingly helpful in explaining the principles that underlie the Women's Diet. In Chapter Eight we turn to the dieting advice of the world's wickedest philosopher, Friedrich Nietzsche.* Writing in the later nineteenth century Nietzsche eagerly looked forward to the time when a new breed of supermen or 'übermensch' would seize power. With the benefit of hindsight, this was not the wisest thing to put in the minds of his readers, but it does give us the Uberdiet.

In the final section of the book we squeeze in four more diets. Two twentieth century philosophers, Franz Kafka and Albert Camus give us the Trial Diet (Chapter Nine) and the Rebel Diet (Chapter Ten). Chapter Eleven briefly considers religious dieting. Finally in Chapter Twelve we go back to Plato, who links dieting to love.

---

* If you go to university you will probably be taught that that the apparent link between Nietzsche and Nazism is 'all his sister's fault.' and that Nietzsche is not really wicked at all. However, if you take the trouble to actually read his books you will quickly find that he *is*.

Meet the Guinea Pigs

When I sketched out my plan for this book, one question bothered me: How on earth was I to get people to read the dieting advice of a dozen or so philosophers without becoming bored? Of course, I myself do not find philosophers boring. In fact, there is nothing I like more than settling down on the bus to work with a copy of Schopenhauer's *Essays* to chortle over. But although quite a few other passengers may also have something to read with them, when I peep over their shoulders I never find anyone else with a work of philosophy in their hands; a few are reading novels, most are engrossed in an article about the latest twist in some reality TV show. Seeing this (and knowing that philosophers like Camus and Kafka use stories to get their message across), my answer to the problem of how to stop people getting bored has been to invent a gang of human guinea pigs to test the diets out.

So who have we got?

Drum Roll

'We have one couple! We have two *gorgeous* ladies! And we have a guy on his tod. So: *Come on out the Guinea Pig Gang!'*

Wild applause
Exuberant saxophone music

The Guinea Pig Gang appear in their best clothes waving and smiling. The couple holds hands. They walk confidently down the steps to stand in a line as the compere moves along the row to introduce them.

Stuart and Wendy

Two brilliant young professionals. Late twenties, Work hard, play hard and holiday in style, but they also eat lots and exercise little and it's starting to show.

Applause

Angela

Forty four. She's been in and out of a number of relationships, but all the time her love handles have been growing, and she's starting to worry about ever holding on to her man.

Enthusiastic applause

Jasmine

Thirty two. She's been overweight ever since she was a little girl. But now she's determined to lose it!

Enthusiastic applause, whoops and wolf whistles

Derek

Forty. Started to get fat when his hair fell out. Divorced. Spends all his holidays in Thailand. Told by his doctor that he should lose weight. Hey feller, it's entirely up to you! We're not here to tell an adult what to do. But if you want to give it a go, you're welcome to join in.

Polite applause

'And now lets get down to business!'

The Guinea Pigs go jogging off the stage waving as they go.

Cheers

Selecting the Guinea Pigs

The greatest philosophical discoveries emerged in the simplest of ways when, in ancient Athens, a small group of people got together and worked their ideas through. It is all described in Plato's *Republic* when Socrates, and five of his friends: Glaucon, Adeimantus, Cephalus, Polemarchus and Thrasymachus sit down and—just by talking to each other—work out the meaning of justice, the basis of human psychology, the best and worst forms of government, and the immortality of the soul. So why not do the same thing with dieting? Perhaps we could try and work out a just diet and the way that dieting is related to our psychology, our government and our soul just by talking it through in a group. And we would lose weight and look great at the same time.

I would be Socrates of course, but I needed to find the other five. So I placed an advertisement with my contact details in the personal section of the local newspaper. The advert read as follows:

> Academic seeks interlocutors for dialectical investigation into the mind-body relationship in dieting. Bergsonian, Cartesian, Hobbesian, Lockean, Hegelian, Marxist, Nietzschean, Platonic and existentialist philosophers will be considered in a series of critical symposia.

No one responded to this announcement and the project might have ended there were it were not for the charismatic Icelandic filmmaker Knud Knudson. Knudson and I had once collaborated on a movie script about a little Japanese girl who grew up in an orphanage and went on to become a brilliant pianist. The film was never made but we kept in touch, and when I mentioned my idea to him he immediately saw its potential. Knudson offered to collaborate with me, I was delighted to agree, and he booked a flight to England.

I had not seen Knudson for some years. Now there were flecks of grey in his beard and the windblown hair had retreated a little from his temples. But he still exuded vitality with his tall, powerful build, keen eyed expression and firm handshake. He reminded me—as he always had—of a Michelangelo figure, though I could never quite remember which one.

With Knudson's assistance and advice I composed a new advert:

Want to lose weight and get on telly?
Leading documentary maker and top philosophy boffin seek five person dieting team for prime time TV series.
Interested? Then send an email and explain why in one sentence.

It did the trick because when I opened my inbox ten people had sent in emails, twice as many as I needed. I still have the ten emails, with the names and the single sentence on my system, and here they are:

> Please accept my application.
> Yours Sincerely,
> Jasmine

> I've got a gap year, and I'm ready to put 100% of my life into this challenge.
> Best,
> Frank Fogg (nickname 'Foggy')

I have a dream that this is my destiny.
Rosemary

I've been abroad and I'd like to meet new people.
Derek

My passion is philosophy and watching documentaries, and yes I could diet.
Yours,
Tansu x

I think it sounds interesting and I'd like to give it a go.
Angela

I am young and confused about my 'identity,'
and this TV show could help me to sort myself out.
Steve

The following two messages came from the same email account:

I need to lose weight.
Wendy

My wife says I need to lose weight.
Stuart

And finally there was this:

You sound like a pair of posh gits, but I'll give it a go. ;-}
Sharon

'What do you think?' asked Knudson. 'Who shall we choose?'

'Well, much of a muchness, really. Hard to know without meeting them.'

'No. You see because I am a film maker and do casting all the time, I already know a lot about these people, and I think I have chosen.'

'You've chosen already? Knud, isn't that a bit premature?'

'No, read them again and you will agree I think: this one, Jasmine, she is boring and no good, that is obvious. But this next one, Foggy in his gap year, with his energy, he is good, like an eager young puppy.'

'Well, yes, the first two do sound different, you're right, but what about the others?'

'This lady Rosemary with her dreams. She is good too, she has masses of character. And she is black, I can tell. But the next one Derek, the man who wants to meet people, he is a no-hoper; this is a TV show not a dating service. Tansu is passionate, mysterious, exotic, full of life and hot gypsy blood. Yes! Angela who says it 'sounds interesting,' is dull—another useless one. Steve is gay; good, we must have at least one. This couple, Wendy and Stuart are colourless and the man is a wimp. No. Sharon is forthright and down to earth, but also she is deeply emotional and archetypically working class. So of course we must have her.'

I was flabbergasted by Knud's Sherlock Holmesish intuition.

'That's incredible Knud! You've worked out all that just from a one line email!'

'But of course, it is my job to know these things.'

'So shall we write to these five...?'

'No, it must be all ten of them, and tell them to bring a change of clothes, because of the tests.'

'Tests?'

'Yes, I have devised some tests for them. There are always tests at the start of these shows, to throw out the bad ones so that the audience can laugh at them.'

'Well, I'm not sure...'

'You are never "sure" Peter, but you will see. And don't worry. As soon as the tests are done, I will go back into the background and just do the filming and you can be in charge again with your philosophy.'

'I suppose there are some advantages to it: I mean they'll start out *not* doing philosophy as a way of *doing* philosophy. It's what we philosophers call dialectics.

' "Dialectics." I like it. That is a good word; I have not heard it before; I will have to look it up. So we are agreed, yes?'

Yes, I agreed to the tests.

The next step was to find a venue. We wanted a low key, homely environment, and as it happened the hall attached to the local church a few streets from my house was perfect. It was a very traditional church hall that hosted cub scout meetings, Bible classes, dancing lessons, and mother and toddler groups. It was bright and airy with a large mirror for the dance class and a whiteboard that I could use while explaining the philosophers.

We called on the rectory next door to the hall and explained to the Reverend Smith that we would be more or less like weight watchers, but with more discussion and less exercise. He was—at that stage—most welcoming and we immediately booked sessions for four months. There was no problem about filming and indeed Edna, the Vicar's wife, seemed rather excited that the church hall was to feature on TV. Sensing this, Knudson quickly worked his Nordic charm upon her and before I knew it, she was offering to make a selection of cakes and pastries for our first meeting.

'They must be soft cakes,' said Knudson firmly. 'No nuts or hard bits.'

'Yes, of course,' said the Vicar's wife, 'allergies, choking, I mean health and safety is so important these days. I remember when we used to give children fish with bones...'

'No fish,' interrupted Knudson irritably, 'we have just agreed on *cake*. Cream, custard: these types of ingredients.'

'I see yes, custard and cream. And chocolate cake, would that be alright?'

Knudson considered this for a few seconds.

'Yes, a soft one.'

The Vicar's wife seemed pleased at this concession; I guessed that she was proud of her chocolate cake.

So that was that. We had our candidates for the diets and we had our venue.

After we had left the vicarage, I joshed Knudson about his seductive impact on the Vicar's wife

'You are wrong. It is you that she wants. For myself it is always the younger ones.'

'She wants *me*?'

'Yes. I am a film director so I know about women. Your woolly jumper and your scholarship are highly attractive to her.'

'Are they really?'

'For sure. It would be a simple matter to adulterate her.'

'You always put things so frankly Knud.'

'When you are directing a film your vision must be clear and your instructions precise. That is also my rule for life.'

Knudson had forgotten to bring his film equipment with him, so with his advice I bought a rather expensive camcorder, and at the appointed hour we arrived at the church hall to find that our ten hopefuls were already there.

Knudson's uncanny abilities meant I already recognised some of the applicants. That young man with the floppy hair and gawky charm could only be Foggy, the tall graceful black lady was surely Rosemary, the beauty smouldering tempestuously in a sheepskin coat was obviously Tansu, the youth wearing the tight white T-shirt was Steve, and the tough looking woman we had met outside the porch smoking a cigarette was Sharon. Standing around in a nondescript kind of way were the other five. We shook hands and I started to clear my throat to make a speech of welcome when Knudson stopped me and passed me the camcorder.

'No. You film. Try and focus on their faces. I will speak to them.'

'OK, Knud. Yes, you go first, sure.'

'Ladies and gentlemen!' said Knudson, 'Welcome, and may I first say congratulations to you all! We have had more than one hundred and fifty applications and it has been a not-easy job deciding who we would invite here. So already you have come an incredibly long way. Because you are now the final ten. So what does this mean?'

Here I focused on Foggy's eager face as he listened intently.

'It means, for five of you, that today is a most important moment because you will be the five chosen ones, the ones who will go through to do the philosophy of dieting!'

There were excited exclamations from the group. Foggy gulped. Tansu's eyes gleamed with excitement. Rosemary took a deep breath and looked determined. Steve looked around to high five with someone and then clapped. Sharon coughed.

Knudson held up his hand, paused and looked serious. Steve immediately looked serious too.

'But for another five of you here, today, in this room, now, this is not the first step, but the last. For today we have some tests. And only half of you can pass these tests. The other half will fail.'

There was a sombre pause, Steve's clean scrubbed face dropped as if he had switched on the TV to be confronted with some hideous event taking place half way across the world, nothing to do with him personally but sobering nonetheless.

'So your chance are 50/50. But I want to say to all of you: Good Luck! OK. First up, we have two teams. No fancy names, just the A Team and the B Team, and we have sorted these in advance so that it is entirely random.'

Knudson got out a list and consulted it.

'For the A Team,' Knudson declared, 'the first member is...Foggy!'

Frank Fogg looked delighted.

'Second, Rosemary!' Rosemary looked surprised and then turned to Foggy like a long lost cousin and hugged him.

'Third, Tansu!' Tansu screamed and hugged them both.

'Fourth, Steve!' Steve made a 'yes' sign with his fist and bounded over to the others, attempting to embrace them all in a kind of rugby scum.

'And fifth... Sharon!' Sharon marched over on her high heels, cool as a cucumber, but with the ghost of a smile playing around her lips.

'OK, and you other five are in the B Team,' said Knudson. 'Now are we ready for your first test?'

'Yes!' called out the A Team. It was at this moment that I had my first vague sensation that there was something awry with Knudson's plan, though I could not yet put my finger on what it was.

Test 1: Teamwork

I live in a town that is almost encircled by a curving brown river, somewhat dirty when you look at it closely but with beautiful woods above its banks. Knudson seemed pleased with this river and wanted to include it in the filming, so for the first test we took our ten hopefuls down there. Using only the detritus and junk that lined the bank each team had to build a raft and float across to the other side. According to Knudson, this test was designed to measure cooperation and teamwork.

The A Team set about things with a will. Foggy was in his element, rushing up and down collecting branches, oil drums, bottles and bits of rope. Tansu and Steve pulled gamely but ineffectually on a large log while Sharon watched them, smoking. She was apparently indifferent to their efforts, yet there was something about her poise that suggested a leopard about to spring. Then with a sudden superb gesture of disdain, she flicked her cigarette into the water, strode over and in a few lithe and powerful movements succeeded in dragging the log up the bank. Steve was amazed.

'Wow. You must do pilates or something?'

'Beer barrels', said Sharon, enigmatically, and lit another cigarette.

Tansu, gorgeous in her skin tight jeans, stepped onto the log and tried to rope-walk along it. Foggy came panting past and Tansu overbalanced. She screamed delightedly as she fell into his arms and the two of them collapsed and rolled playfully on the ground. Steve jumped up and down and clapped.

Soon the A team's raft was done. Rosemary, erect at the tiller like a Nubian queen, gave the orders as the others crouched beneath her and paddled furiously with makeshift implements. Foggy threw the 'grappling hook' at a tree; it caught and they had made it. There were cheers and hugs on the far bank.

The B Team, who already seemed to sense that they were going to be dumped, trooped listlessly down to the water. Stuart and Wendy collected a small pile of wood and then stood looking at it helplessly. They seemed to be waiting for the raft to build itself. Jasmine ('my clothes might get dirty'), and Angela ('I don't want Weil's disease') did nothing whatsoever, they just spent their time chatting together on the bank taking little notice of what was going on. Derek ostentatiously walked across the bridge.

Test 2: The Will to Win

Back in the church hall the Vicar's wife had been across from the rectory and had set out a table full of buns, cream tarts, custard pies, small delicate fairy cakes and a large chocolate cake thickly coated in cocoa butter icing. The food was tempting, but before anyone could launch into it, Knudson stopped them. The next test, he said, would measure your will to win. The food was not to be eaten, rather everyone was to throw it at each other.

Once again I had a nagging feeling that something was not quite right. I still did not know what, but I now sensed that the problem lay with the A Team. This, however, hardly seemed fair as they responded so enthusiastically to the new challenge. Rosemary and Sharon hurled pies energetically at one other. Their battle was relentless, almost vicious, yet somehow you realised that they *respected* each other and, through the medium of pie throwing, were starting to like one another too, exhibiting in microcosm the success of Britain's multiethnic and multicultural society. Foggy and Tansu laughed blissfully as they slavered each other in the chocolate cake. Steve hovered brightly on the edges not quite sure how to join in.

The B Team did not really participate. Angela, Jasmine and Wendy had simply walked out of the room; Stuart and Derek were still in there, but only because they were, contrary to the rules, eating the pies. Steve walked over to them and with a slightly nervous laugh made as if to pitch a cream tart at Derek. Derek scowled and showed his fist. Steve backed off.

Test 3: Leadership

Dark chocolate brown stains still smeared the floor where Foggy and Tansu had wrestled, but with the help of the A Team girls and the contents of the broom cupboard the rest of the church hall was now more or less clean. The A Team had changed their clothes and looked tired but happy, their eyes alight for whatever might come next. The B Team looked somewhat resentful.

'For the leadership test one of you will be wrapped in toilet paper,' began Knudson, when Derek butted in.

'We're not doing any more of your fucking tests and that's final.'

There was a shocked silence. Then Knudson responded coldly but politely.

'Can I ask you why not?'

'Because this is a farce: we're leaving.'

'OK. But wait a minute please, since you have enjoyed our hospitality today, and our pies, yes'—Knudson looked pointedly at Derek's paunch—'some of you several pies!'

It was then that the vague feeling of unease that had been troubling me all day hit me like a bolt of lightning.

'You will at least listen when I announce the result?' Knudson continued.

I looked at the B Team, and then I looked at the A Team. Oh my goodness, what a fool I had been! How *could* I not have noticed before?

'So I need a quick discussion with my fellow judge,' said Knudson.

The A Team was expectant and on edge, the B Team muttering indignantly. Knudson turned to me.

It has been said that the philosophy of dieting group got off on a bad footing, and that had things been different at the beginning, they might have turned out better in the end. I think, therefore, that it is important to place on the record exactly what happened so that people can make up their own minds. The transcript below is taken verbatim from my camcorder, which I had placed on the table and which was left running for the entire time. It begins with my final conversation with Knud Knudson a few seconds after I had realised what the problem was, and it ends with the announcement of the winners of the competition.

TRANSCRIPT 1

KNUD: So?

PETER: (whispers) Knud, I've got to talk to you urgently.

KNUD: Sure, I will just read out the result otherwise the fat lot are going to leave.

PETER: (whispers) Wait Knud, that's the point.

KNUD: [in loud voice ignoring PETER] Ladies and Gentlemen. The judges have reached their decision, and I am going to open this envelope and read it out to you.

KNUD: (tears open envelope)

THE A TEAM: (clasp hands in excitement)

THE B TEAM: (roll their eyes at the charade)

KNUD: OK. I can now announce...

PETER: (holds KNUD'S arm) Wait Knud!

KNUD: (To teams) Hold on please ladies and gentlemen: judges' conference. (To PETER: [irritably]) What?

PETER: (whispers) I've worked out what's wrong with them!

KNUD: Wrong with who?

PETER: The one's we're going to select, the A Team: Foggy, Rosemary, Tansu, Steve and Sharon (glances at A TEAM who are looking on anxiously).

KNUD: Well, What?

PETER: None of them are fat! Only the B Team are fat.

KNUD: Fat?

PETER: No, and they need to be, because we're *dieting*.

KNUD: Fat? What is 'fat?' Compared to someone who is starving, they are fat.

PETER: Yes, but not fat enough.

KNUD: Peter, you gone a little crazy. You don't need to be fat to go on a diet!

PETER: Yes you do, because otherwise, what's the point?

KNUD: (increasingly loudly) So what are you saying? You want me to choose the other ones just because they are overweight?

PETER: Well, yes.

KNUD: [not making any effort to lower his voice] But I thought you agreed that they're a bunch of no-hopers without personality?

PETER: I know I did, but...

KNUD: (temples starting to throb) And now! This is most ridiculous.

PETER: I'm sorry Knud.

KNUD: (exploding with anger) No! (To teams) Please ladies and gentlemen. I owe you, or half of you, an apology. (Turning to the A TEAM) You, the ones who have been in the river and doing the food fight so well. You have been magnificent. But despite all of that, my partner here, Mr Philosopher, he says that you are all to be kicked out, and that we go with this other lot (indicating the B TEAM). Even though they are useless. But that does not matter. Because, as you can see, they all have big tummies.

(Consternation in the A TEAM: FOGGY looks confused, STEVE horrified, TANSU furious, SHARON icy, ROSEMARY tragic.)

KNUD: Yes, I share your disquiet. Can I be permitted to say one thing? I have seen enough of you today to know this: you are all beautiful human beings. And together we could have gone on a fantastic journey. But no. According to our philosopher friend in the woolly jumper, it is you who are kicked out. Well, I tell you one thing: I go too. I quit Peter. I leave you with your fatties.

(KNUD, STEVE, SHARON, ROSEMARY, TANSU and FOGGY all leave.)

(DEREK, JASMINE, WENDY, STUART and ANGELA stand and stare at them go. They look perplexed, not quite sure what is going on.)

PETER: (to B Team) Well, congratulations!

So there it is. That was how the Guinea Pig Gang were selected (for of course the Guinea Pig Gang are one and the same as the B Team) and as I say, I leave you to make your own mind up about it. This whole sorry affair with Knudson and his absurd tests was nothing to do with dieting philosophy at all, and I mention it only because it caused problems later on. However, from the moment Knudson flounced out of the room the philosophising began, as I introduced the Guinea Pigs to the philosophical concepts of logic and of dialectics.

Logic and Dialectics

If we are going to understand the weight-loss suggestions of our philosophers we must learn a little jargon first. So we will begin with a familiar word, 'logic,' and compare it to a less familiar one, 'dialectics.' Logic and dialectics are two very different ways of getting to the truth. Logic is a way of working things out where you *start with a simple truth* (or what you hope is the truth) *and then build on it to reach a more complicated truth.* This is quite different from dialectics which means *telling lies at the beginning in order to reach the truth in the end.* When Knudson and the A team had left, I had a choice of using logic or dialectics on the Guinea Pigs. If I had chosen logic I would have told them the simple truth from the start: that without Knudson's media contacts the prospect of a TV documentary was finished. I did not do that. Why not? *Because it would not have helped them to reach the more complicated truth of how to lose weight.* Only by lying could I help them.

And I had to lie quickly. We were left in the church hall, five Guinea Pigs and me, and they were obviously on the point of leaving too.

'What's going to happen now about us being on telly?' asked Stuart anxiously.

'Yes. I mean, if Knud's gone and he's the film maker there's no point in doing this diet thing is there?' said Jasmine.

'Oh well,' said Angie, 'anyone want a cup of coffee?'

At this point, I *could* have said something like: 'Get your priorities straight! Yes, the documentary has been abandoned, but that's not why you need to be here. You don't need to get on TV, you need to lose weight!' That would have been true and logical, but it also would have been counterproductive. The Guinea Pigs were already suspicious and disgruntled, and if I had said something like that they would have taken offence and left. In short, it was useless trying to persuade the Guinea Pigs to stay with logic. So I used dialectics instead. First I tapped my camcorder, which was still running, and explained that I would be continuing to film them with it. Then I deliberately switched the camera off.

'Can you keep a secret?' I asked. They could.

'Knud hasn't really packed in. That was all an act. Really he's taken the other group off somewhere else and will be filming them there.'

The Guinea Pigs immediately believed this. Derek indeed had already 'guessed as much.' But it also made them very curious, firing questions at me.

'So we're sort of competing against the other team?'

'Yes.'

'Where has Knud taken them?'

'I can't say. That's a secret.'

'Some tropical island I bet!'

I gasped and raised my eyebrows, then pursed my lips tight.

'Yeah, I guessed that much too,' said Derek shrewdly. 'So where're you taking *us*?'

'Ah, that I *can* tell you. We're staying here.'

There was disappointment at that news, but there was also satisfaction among the Guinea Pigs that at least they were still going to be on telly. Perhaps they also hoped that at a later stage they might also get to go to Knud's tropical island. By lying to them, therefore, I had prepared the way for the Guinea Pigs to begin to learn the profound *truths* of philosophy, as well as to lose weight. Later, when the time was ripe, I planned to tell them that they were not in fact going to be on TV at all, by which time it would not matter to them. *That* was dialectics.

Dear Mrs Smith,
Thank you very much for the cakes and things. It was most kind of you to make them and we all really enjoyed them.

Best Wishes

Peter

Part I
The Nice Philosophers

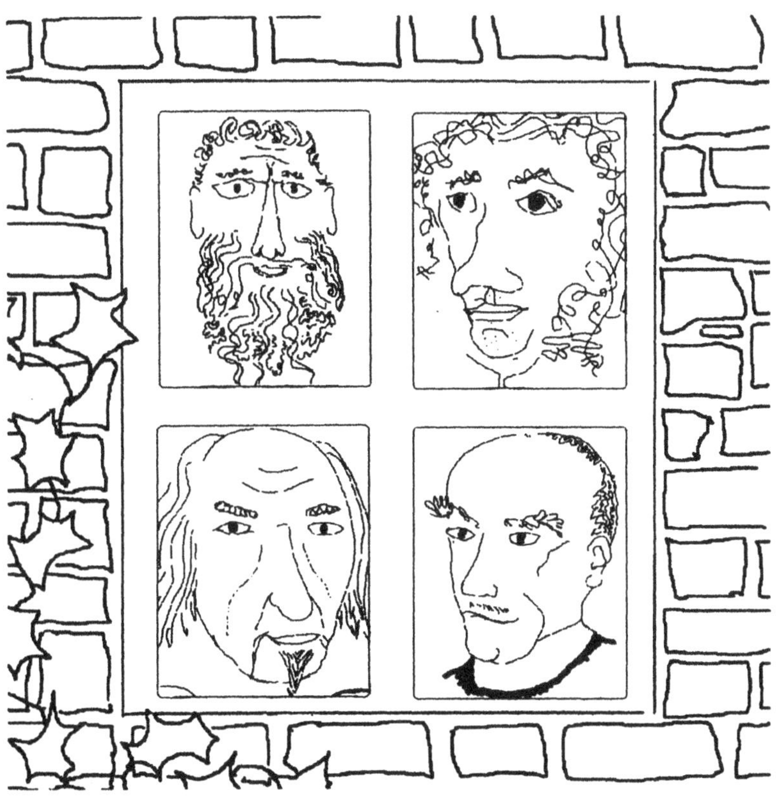

Chapter 1
Bergson's Laughter Diet

which explains why, if you want to be serious about losing weight, you first have to laugh about it.

It is a sad fact that overweight people often become figures of fun. Amongst children, and sometimes even amongst adults, simply being different from what is seen as normal has been a cause of laughter. And leading the list are people who are overweight. Since time immemorial kids have laughed at other kids for being plump. Comic figures from John Falstaff to Oliver Hardy are overweight. We have to face it; there is something funny about being fat.

Now I want to make it absolutely 100% clear that laughing at other people because they are overweight is wrong. It is not quite as bad as, say, laughing at someone who has learning difficulties, but it is still pretty bad. It's nasty, it's immature, it's a bit like being racist, and we are not going to go there.[*]

But there is one person who is fat who you *can* laugh at.

Yourself.

Laughing at others is cruel. But laughing at yourself is liberating. This, at least, is Henri Bergson's idea in a little book he wrote about laughter. Bergson says that if you can laugh about being fat it will make you feel better about yourself and it will start to make you feel free. Sounds good? Then let's try it.

The great thing about this dieting philosophy is it's very easy to do, and if you're at home, you can actually start

* At least, not until Chapter Eight.

immediately. In fact, Bergson's laughter diet is so easy that it can be reduced to a simple three point plan. And here it is:

1. Take your clothes off.
2. Stand in front of a full length mirror.
3. Laugh.

Go on, give it a go right now. If you don't laugh straight away, get your tummy to wobble and say 'Hello jelly baby!' And no peeking at the next paragraph until after you're done!

Given it a try? Good. And if you could really laugh at yourself, that is fantastic. But when I did it with the Guinea Pig Gang that's not what happened.

We were assembled in the kitchen of the church hall, and took in turns to go through and stand in front of the mirror in the main room. Wendy and her husband Stuart volunteered to go in together first and this broke the ice. Unfortunately though, and despite my instructions, when they laughed they laughed at each other rather than at themselves.

Angela went in front of the mirror next and she laughed, but I could tell that it wasn't a *proper* laugh. She laughed in an anxious, forced kind of way, like she didn't really mean it.

Then Jasmine went in front of the mirror, and started to cry.

At first I misinterpreted the noise. I had been a bit disappointed that the other three hadn't been laughing in the right way, so when I began to hear snuffles from Jasmine I was really excited.

'Superb. Jasmine's laughing. Bergson is *so* smart!' I thought. But as the noise went on I realised that it was, unmistakably, crying that was coming though the door, not laughter. Then Jasmine started sobbing uncontrollably.

I didn't know what to do.

Henri Bergson at work thinking

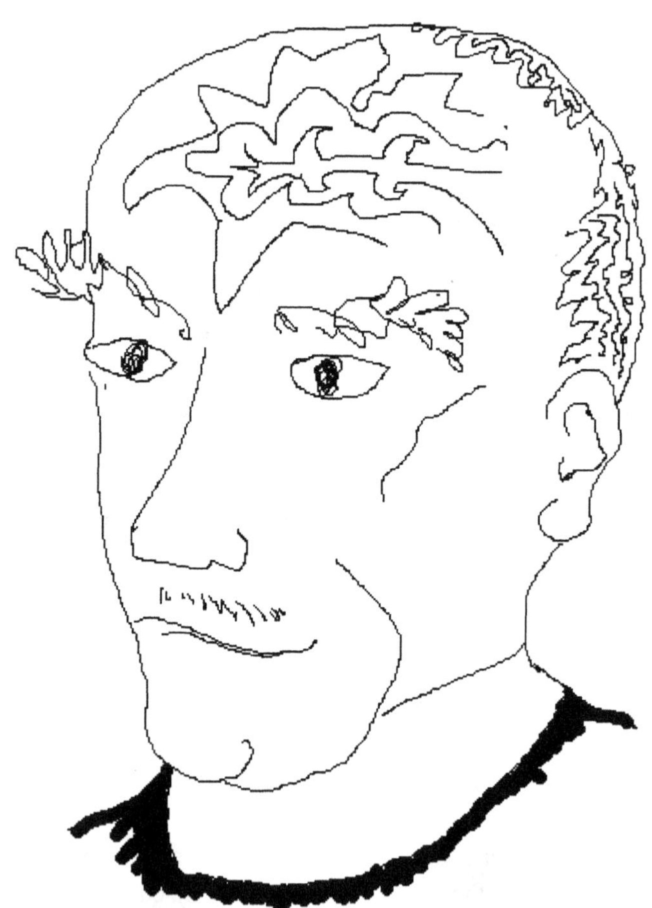

Angela went into the hall—she had already made friends with Jasmine—and eventually things quietened down. Jasmine came out red eyed but OK, and we all sat down in the kitchen and had a cup of tea. When I felt she was ready, I asked Jasmine if she could tell us about what had happened in there.

'I took my clothes off, and I was standing there looking at myself, and at all the fat on me. And I'm thinking: 'Laugh? How can I laugh about this?' I mean, like my body is my nightmare. It's spoilt just about everything for me. You know, I'm getting older and, basically, being fat has ruined my life. All the guys, you know guys that I liked. Well, I mean, none of them's ever wanted to go out with me, not properly like we're dating. And it's not just that either. I get so out of breath I can't do anything. Like one of my friends from school, we've kept in touch, and she did this incredible outdoor thing in Scotland, and sent me the photos; they looked so amazing. But, it just made me feel trapped, because, I mean I get tired just walking round the shopping centre. And that's why, when I saw myself, and all my, fat, I, well…'

Jasmine started to gulp and sniff and Angela came in protectively.

'Listen Jasmine, I think you look great. I really do. And hey, you've done stuff; you've rescued a cat from the shelter; you've started to paint your kitchen pink, and you're going to do the bedroom…'

As Angela comforted her friend, I felt a bit stuck. At one level, I could appreciate what she was doing. It was a warm, human reaction to reassure Jasmine and to try and stop her from feeling upset. But at another level, I was annoyed. This was the first proper meeting of the Guinea Pigs and already it seemed like session was turning into some kind of support group. Dieting philosophy is not about sympathy and hugs and this was not where I wanted the Guinea Pigs to go, so I broke in and stopped it with a question from out of the blue.

'Jasmine, what's your favourite book?'

'Book? I read a book about Princess Diana once. But usually I prefer magazines.'

'Fine, what's your favourite magazine then?'

'Cosmopolitan.'

'OK so you want to be a cosmo girl, and being fat's stopped you?'

'Yes, I guess so.'

'I'll tell you one of my favourite books. It's called *'The Diary of Anne Frank.'*[*]

Angela pursed her lips and Wendy and Stuart looked puzzled. But Jasmine took it in her stride. In fact, she broke into a chuckle.

'Oh yeah, I know that one, I saw the movie.'

Actually Jasmine didn't know that one. She was getting mixed up with *The Diary of Bridget Jones*. Of course, I could see why, because there are a lot of laughs about dieting in it, but before I could correct her, everyone started talking about how true to life it was and how they'd felt the same way as Bridget about their weight. And then Derek, who had wandered in late, said that to be honest he really liked Renée Zellweger's bottom (she played Bridget Jones in the movie), and we all got diverted into talking about our favourite

---

[*] Anne Frank's *Diary of a Young Girl* was written while she and her family, who were Jewish, attempted to hide from the Nazis in Amsterdam during the Second World War. The diary ends abruptly when the family is betrayed and Anne is sent to her death in a concentration camp.

bottoms and laughing about that. Then the Vicar's wife arrived, with some homemade teacakes, to thank me for my note. After that the Guinea Pigs tried to quiz me about the island where Knudson had taken the A Team, and it ended up that I never did let on about what I had meant.

Angela had caught on though. She didn't say anything at the time, but underneath it had made her really angry and later, after the others had gone, she confronted me about it.

'That thing about Anne Frank. I know what you were trying to say: that just because Jasmine's not had a terrible accident, or been mutilated, or hunted by Nazis or whatever, that she's making a big fuss about nothing. Peter, I'll tell you what I think about that comment. I think it was cheap.'

Then she turned and left.

Angela was right. That was, more or less, what I had wanted to say to Jasmine. And she was right about something else too, it *was* cheap, because the way that I'd put things wasn't going to make Jasmine feel any better about herself and it certainly wasn't going to make her laugh. I thought long and hard about this, and at our next session, I did something different. But first, let me try and defend myself by explaining why Jasmine did not really having anything to be sad about, at least in terms of the philosophical distinction between tragedy and comedy.

Tragedy and Comedy

When Jasmine looked in the mirror, her mistake was thinking that the excess fat on her body was a tragedy. Actually it was a comedy. To put it brutally, the fact that Jasmine thought she was locked into some kind of tragic destiny just because she was overweight would have made philosophers laugh. And though I had gone about it the wrong way, I had wanted

Jasmine to laugh at the idea too, because once she could realise the absurdity of thinking that being fat is tragic she could start to do something about it.

We all know that tragedy means something sad and comedy means something happy. But when philosophers like Aristotle or Hegel or Marx use these words they mean a little bit more. To explain this we can compare a couple of *abc* lists.

The ABC of Tragedy

A tragedy occurs when:

(a) something *very bad* happens

that is

(b) *inevitable* (there is no way of avoiding it, it is your *fate* or *destiny*)

and

(c) *is not your fault*

The ABC of Comedy

A comedy occurs when:

(a) something *only a little bit bad* happens

that

(b) would have been *easy to avoid* if you hadn't made a *simple mistake*

and

(c) *is your own fault.*

When we read Anne Frank's diary we are reading a tragedy; her family's desperate effort to escape infinitely more powerful enemies makes the dreadful outcome more or less inevitable, and obviously not Anne's fault. When Jasmine looked at her overweight body, she thought she was looking at another tragedy. But was she? Remember, something which makes you feel sad, even very sad, does not mean that it automatically qualifies as a tragedy. Let's go back to our *abc* of tragedy and work it out.

(a) Is being overweight very bad. Jasmine thought the answer to this was Yes, but philosophically speaking the answer is No—I'll come back to this a bit later and explain why.

(b) Is being overweight inevitable? Is there no way of avoiding it? Is it your fate or destiny? Jasmine thought Yes. Actually the answer is No. All you need to do to lose weight is eat less food and do more exercise, and this can hardly be said to be impossible.

(c) Is being overweight your own fault? Jasmine thought No. Because she had been fat ever since she was little, this might have been true, once. But *now*, as an adult, Jasmine is responsible for her own weight: the answer is Yes.

Now, let's move on to comedy and work our way backwards from c to a.

(c) Is being overweight your own fault? Yes.

(b) Is being overweight easy to avoid if you don't make a simple mistake?

Yes!

What is that simple mistake?

Thinking that being overweight is tragic.

If you think being overweight means you are caught in a tragedy, it means you think you can't do anything about it, when really *you can*. To lose weight, you have to change that mindset. That's why it's so important to try and laugh about it.

(a) Is being overweight just a little bit bad?

Yes. It hardly counts as being bad at all.

The Comedy of Othello

Angela had seemed so cross that I was worried that she was going to drop out of the Guinea Pig Gang, so I called on her with a bunch of flowers and asked if I could explain what I'd been trying to do. She agreed to let me in and we sat in her kitchen while I took her through the difference between tragedy and comedy. I explained it using a piece of paper with a chart on it like this:

Comparing Tragedy and Comedy

	Tragedy	**Comedy**
How bad?	Very Bad	Not too Bad
Inevitable?	Yes	No
Your own fault?	No	Yes

Angela thought about it and said:

'I can see where you're coming from and I can see what you are trying to say: being fat is comic not tragic. But no way is Jasmine's life a comedy. She's unhappy about her weight; how it makes her look; how it makes her feel; how it prevents her forming relationships. And that's not funny. Jasmine said that because of being fat she felt she'd had a bit of a rotten life. OK, I agree that she may have made mistakes. I agree that perhaps it didn't have to be that way. *But it was.* And she's suffered because of it.'

I started to reply by talking about Anne Frank again, but Angela broke in.

'Of course things could be much, much worse. But I still think you can call being fat a tragedy. You might have read Hegel and Aristotle, but I've read *Othello.*[*] He made mistakes, did things wrong, and the mess he created was his own fault. But still, nobody calls it 'The Comedy of Othello.' It was a *tragedy.*'

When Angela mentioned *Othello* it caught me off guard.

'Hey! *I'm* the one with the PhD,' I thought. 'You're just one of the Guinea Pigs.' (Perhaps it was then that I started to realise that there was more to Angela than met the eye—something that, in the end, I learned about all of them.) And it wasn't just an educated comment, it was a really good one too. Because it made me see why Angela and I were disagreeing with each other: we had been arguing about different things. Angela was talking about the *past.* I was talking about the *future.*

'Angela,' I said, 'my Dad used to tell me that "today is the first day of the rest of your life." And that's true no matter how old you are. You're right; *Othello* is a story that *ends* in tragedy. But Jasmine's life, your life, the lives of all the Guinea Pigs, they're not ending: every day, every moment, they're just *beginning.* OK. We both know that Jasmine's always been fat and it has made her unhappy. And maybe this is a tragedy. But we also know, at least I know, that it doesn't have to be that way, that her future can be different. Jasmine's not *fated* to be fat. She can lose the weight. It's not that hard and it won't take that long. Once she gets going, she'll start to notice the difference in a week. And that's not very bad. It's not even a bit bad. Actually, it's kind of exciting.'

Angela was looking puzzled at this, so I added a bit more.

---

[*] A play by William Shakespeare.

'Let's put it another way. I think that Jasmine has got her past and her future *mixed up*. When she looks in the mirror, she sees her past *and* her future as well. That's her mistake. It's a simple mistake. And when she realises that her image in the mirror is *not* her future, I think, I hope, that she might not feel so unhappy.'

'You mean that you sort of get into the habit of thinking "being fat, that's just the way I am and nothing's going to change it. I'm just going to be like that forever"?'

'Yes. And of course it's true that nothing can change the past. But the future is down to you. You are free to do what you want in the future.'

'So is that where Bergson's freedom idea comes in? He was saying that you laugh about being fat when you realise you are free to do something about it?'

'That's part of it, yes. And the other reason you laugh is that you realise you've been doing this dumb thing: imagining that you're like a robot or something and you can't control yourself when you eat. And that's because you've got the future and the past all mixed up together.'

Angela thought for a bit.

'You know Pete, It's not just Jasmine you're talking about. It's me too. When I look in the mirror, that's what I think: that being fat's a tragedy. And of course, it's not.

Then she laughed.

Yes!

Over the next few weeks, The Guinea Pigs and I worked on Bergson's laughter diet. We had a lot of fun, got to know each other, and by the end of it the 'Pigs' were all laughing properly. Laughing may not be enough on its own to lose weight, but it is a vital preliminary to the success of any other diet. So, now that you have read this chapter, I hope you can see why I've written the book in a way that tries to be light-hearted. At first you might have thought this shows that I am not serious about getting you to lose weight. In fact it shows exactly the opposite: fun and laughter are an essential first step to the philosophy of dieting.

The Laughter Diet in a Nutshell

1. Take your clothes off and stand before the mirror.
2. Remember that you are not a victim of a cruel and unjust fate. You are free.
3. Laugh

Sources

Aristotle, *Poetics*
H. Bergson, *Laughter*
H. Bergson, *Essai sur les données immédiates de la conscience* (Time and free will: the immediate data of consciousness)
GWF Hegel, *Philosophy of Right*
K. Marx, *The Eighteenth Brumaire of Louis Bonaparte*

Dear Edna,
Thank you <u>so much</u> for the teacakes. That was a wonderful surprise for us. And thank you again for the marvellous custard pies and cream pies and the chocolate cake the other day. We absolutely <u>loved</u> them.

You are a very talented woman Edna!

Warmest Good Wishes
Peter

Chapter 2
Plato's Diet of Pigs

Plato's first diet is easy to follow. Don't be put off by the 'pigs' in the title; it just means that the diet is close to nature.

Plato engaging in dialectics

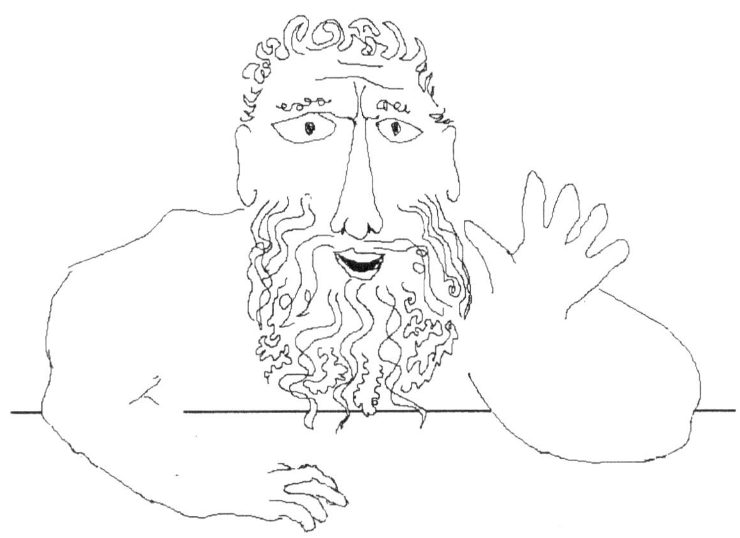

I was sitting on the bench next to the bronze statue of Albert Einstein in Washington DC. It is a wonderful place to visit and on that day, it was beautiful spring weather, people from all over the United States and some, like me, from other parts of the world were walking beneath the blossoming cherry trees of the 'Mall.' From the classical colonnades of the Capitol down to the Lincoln Memorial where Martin Luther King once stood, the Washington Mall is a monument to human achievement In the museums lining the strip, the history of progress in painting, music, and all forms of technology is revealed. This includes the history of flight, with one of Charles Lindbergh's planes suspended from the roof of the Smithsonian. Across the Potomac, beneath an eternal flame is the grave of that great President who launched America on its race to the Moon, nearby the grave of Robert Peary, the first man to have successfully pretended to have reached the North Pole. It was uplifting to be there. To what heights had we soared! I felt that I had arrived at the original 'hall of fame,' that in Washington was collected the most outstanding scientists, artists, engineers and heroes, those who had inspired humanity with their tremendous creativity and intellect, their physical and moral courage, their outstanding chutzpah. They all came together, here, on this spring day. It was as though I was sat atop a great pyramid at the very apex of western civilisation.

But if civilisation had advanced so far I could not help but wonder why it was that so many people were so fat? I said that people were 'walking' up and down along the Mall on that spring day, but this was not strictly accurate, a surprisingly high proportion of them were waddling. If I had switched on the 'documentary' camera it would have been easy to focus on one overweight person after another: overweight ladies going in to the office, a rotund tracksuited street dancer, a crocodile of podgy school children. Surely, I thought, this was backwards. Why was it that the more our civilisation moved forwards, the fatter we all become? What kind of 'progress' is that? As we become more and more civilised, shouldn't we become *less* fat? I started counting people who appeared to me to be overweight, incredibly it seemed to be about a third of them. If you want to take a break from reading try searching 'percentage overweight' on the internet and the evidence of my eyes will be borne out by the figures. You will find that about 24% of white people, 29% percent of Hispanic people and 34% of black people in the USA are not just overweight, but *obese*, and the numbers are rising all the time. 'Is it our fast food?' I wondered. 'Our cars? Sitting in front of the television?' These explanations seemed a bit pat, a bit easy: no, there was surely something else going on. But what?

Pondering on these matters I wandered down the steps into the Museum of African Art. The tribal artefacts and the photographs of dancing, costumes, and rituals were all very interesting, although it was difficult to know quite what was going on. Tribal society remains mysterious in many ways. One thing, however, stood out like a sore thumb. Whatever else they may have been up to, the tribespeople of Africa were certainly not spending their time getting fat. In fact they had beautiful bodies. So what exactly was the difference between them and us? Could we, perhaps learn something from them?

It came to me in a flash; the contrast that I had seen that day, between the overweight people all around me and the photos of the tribespeople. Two thousand five hundred years ago, Plato had noticed *exactly the same thing*. Tribal people, Plato realised, were invariably fit and healthy, while all around him in Athens, the cradle of western civilisation, his fellow citizens were becoming overweight. Now obviously you cannot blame this on cars and MacDonalds and TV because there weren't any back then. The source of people becoming overweight must lie in something deeper, *something that Ancient Athens and present day Washington DC have in common*, something that lies at the very heart of western civilisation.

What is that *thing*? I mean the thing about western civilisation that is making us become more and more overweight? Plato had an extraordinary and audacious answer to this question, one that can shock us even today. But before I tell you, why not guess what he might have said? And if you want a clue, think carefully about what it is that makes both Athens and Washington DC famous cities.

Have you had a guess? OK. I'm going to put my TV-compere-voice on:

Drum roll

Plato's answer to the question of why more and more of us in the west are becoming overweight can be summarised in a single word:

Drum roll get louder

Democracy

Clash of cymbals!

That's right. According to Plato democracy is making us fat. You may think that this is crazy but that is what he said. We're going to work our why he said it and, if you agree with me that he's at least half right, we will start to think about what we can do about it. But first, let us pause to consider that odd statistic that black people in the US are, on average, even more likely to be overweight than white people, with Hispanics somewhere in between. From Plato's perspective, the reason for this may be connected with the rise of democracy. Only since the civil rights campaign have minorities in America been incorporated into democracy as equal citizens, and they are making up for lost time.

As soon as I remembered Plato, the reason why we westerners are fat and getting fatter all the time began falling into place. In a democracy we are equal, so no one is better than you are, and as long as you obey the law, no one has the right to boss you around. Nor is their opinion any better than yours. Democracy *inspires* you with ideas of freedom, or as Plato puts it, it *infects* you with them. In a democracy you think: 'I am free and that means I can do what I like; no one can tell me what to do. If I want to do it, I am going to do it.' In a democracy we are told: Follow your dreams! Reach for the stars!

Now this is great politically, but it has a big dietary downside. It means that you are so used to being free and doing what you desire that when it comes to food, you just cannot stop yourself. In a democracy we are free to do what we like, we have all these choices and want to do all kinds of things, desiring all of them. One of the things we desire is food, food of all kinds, food in great quantities. Our desire for food is easy to satisfy—or so it seems. However, many of our other desires are not. We may have the chance, theoretically, to be great scientists and artists and heroes, but most of us never will be because we are not clever enough, or not creative enough, or not brave enough. So we eat lots instead. Then, of course, we find that the more we eat the more we want to eat, and start to gain weight. But we desire to be slim. So we swap back and forth between eating too much and going on strict diets. If Plato could have looked into the future to see that there was a huge diet industry catering for this, he would not have been at all surprised. In fact, Plato explains that people whose weight yo-yos up and down as they go on and off diets are *typical* of a democracy; we can never stick with a diet for long because our desires are always telling us to do something else.

Living in the great civilisation that was Athens, Plato saw the results of democracy all around him as his friends over ate while lounging around on cushions.

An Athenian

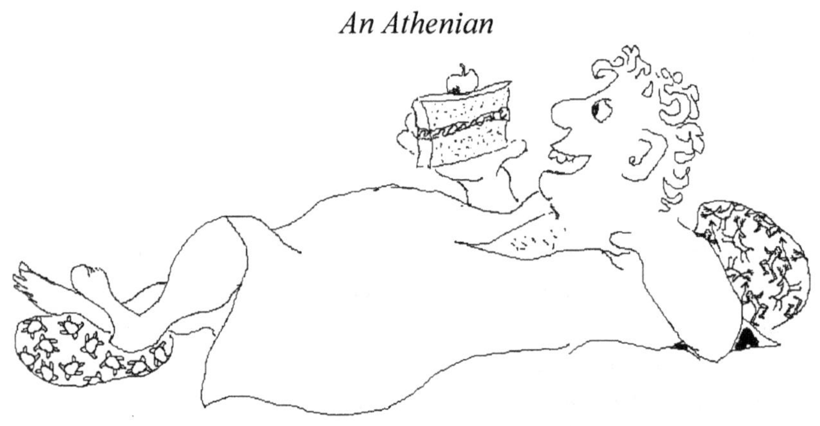

This became a serious military problem when democratic Athens went to war with Sparta, because in Sparta, which was not at all democratic, everyone had superb iron stomachs. Sparta was a much smaller state than Athens, but still in the end the Athenians lost the war. Today too, democracy is at war, and while I do not want to push the parallels too far, one of the ways in which the prisoners captured in the tribal areas of Afghanistan have been mistreated in Guantanamo is by being fed on rich fatty foods, to make them as overweight as the average American. There is, perhaps, some intuition that the lean physique of the enemies of democracy is itself a kind of threat.

Tremendously excited at Plato's insight into why westerners are overweight, I rushed over to Kramer's, bought a copy of *The Republic*, jotted down a quick translation of one of the key passages and returned to my prearranged rendez vous on the Mall. Just as I arrived, Guinea Pigs Stuart and Wendy turned up brandishing a photo of themselves in front of the Whitehouse. They were shaking hands with a cardboard cut out of Barack Obama.

Stuart and Wendy were on holiday in the USA to celebrate the death of Stuart's uncle, who had left his nephew a fortune in his will, and they had taken me with them. Wendy, Stuart and I had hit it off tremendously well when we were practicing the laughter diet, so much so that I had quickly become a sort of father figure to them. Nothing was more natural, therefore, than that when they went on holiday I should come too. I should add that Stuart and Wendy had not paid me to come with them, but were merely financing the necessary expenses of the trip such as flights and hotels, etc. And, to be honest, I only went on holiday with them because I felt protective of them. They had inherited an endless stream of money but neither of them had the faintest idea how to keep hold of it, and they were naïve and easy to take in. Stuart, with his friendly moon face, and Wendy, with her doe eyed Indian squaw look, reminded me of children not quite understanding how the world worked. Indeed, when they initially invited me to come, their idea was to go first to Disneyland in California and then to Disney World in Florida. It took quite a bit of persuading to get them to drop this childish itinerary and instead to take a more sensible adult trip to Washington DC, San Francisco and New York.

A Spartan

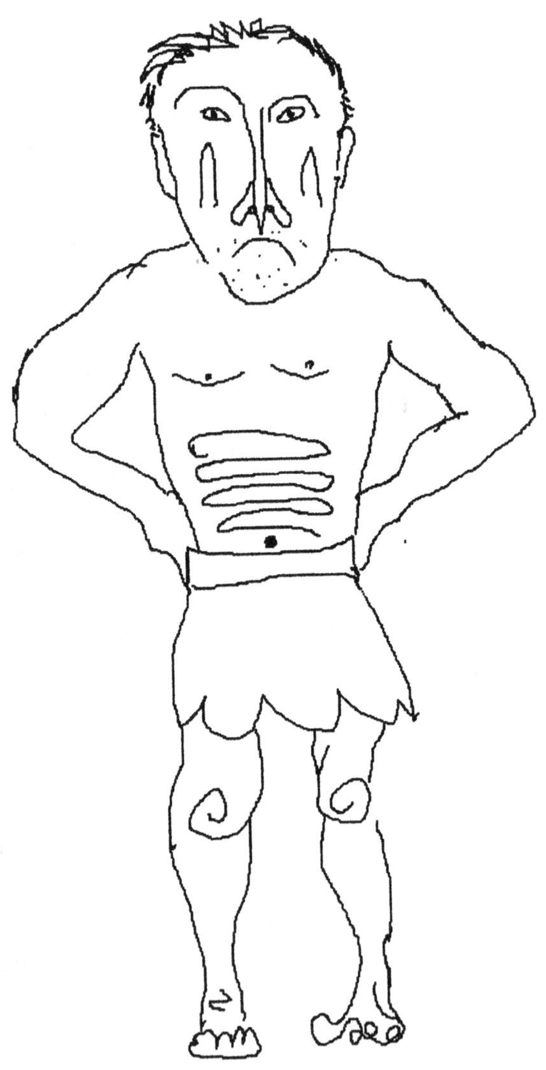

When I told Stuart and Wendy that they were overweight because they lived in a democracy they were, at first, incredulous. I waved *The Republic* at them and told them what Plato had said: Democracy makes you fat, it makes you unhealthy, it makes you pass wind a lot.

'No way,' giggled Stuart. 'Philosophers don't talk like that!'

'Yes they do,' I replied, translating the passage where Plato points out that living in a democracy makes us 'fart like a smelly pond.'

'Well maybe democracy is something to do with it,' admitted Wendy thoughtfully. 'I mean, we both always vote, even in local elections.' Then suddenly she was filled with hope.

'Peter! Do you think that if we stop voting then we will lose weight?'

'That's a good question Wendy,' I replied, 'and I only wish it was that simple, but unfortunately it's not. Democracy is about much more than voting. It's about your rights and your freedoms. You see, whether you vote or not you are living in a democracy all the time. You don't even think about it and take it for granted because you think that it is "natural" to be free and do whatever you choose. And mostly that is a very good thing. It is just for dieting that it's a real problem.'

'Well what can we do then?'

In reply, I showed Stuart and Wendy the passage I had translated, from *The Republic*. I explained to them how Plato (in the mouth of Socrates) was really worried about a brother of his, who was a bit of a couch potato and who was always snacking. To help his brother, Plato/Socrates did not just tell him bluntly and logically that he needed to get a grip and start losing weight. Instead he approached the problem dialectically through a story in which he tactfully invented an imaginary village where everyone followed an excellent diet, and how this made them really healthy with super marital relationships and long happy lives. I continued that Plato's brother had been inspired by this wonderful description to try the diet for himself, and how it had really worked, and turned him around. Finally I asked Stuart and Wendy if they would try the diet, just for a week, to see how they got on with it. Of course they both said that they would, though as things turned out only one of them did. But I am jumping ahead. Let us first see what Plato has to say.

Plato's Diet

In Book Two of *The Republic* Plato (via Socrates) describes a simple but fulfilling way of life to some of his friends, including Plato's couch potato brother, a young man named Glaucon:

> 'In the summer everyone in the village goes around naked with bare feet. But then in the winter they wrap up all furry and snug. They bake bread and cakes from wheat and barley and serve them on plates of reeds. They all get together, grown-ups and youngsters, feasting and singing to the gods. They lie around with garlands of leaves in their hair drinking wine. And of course they have plenty of great sex. But they're careful not to have too many babies, because they don't want to end up making themselves poor or having to start fighting for space.'

At this point Glaucon interrupted:

'Hey! You can't just have them eating bread on its own!'

'You're right,' I replied. 'I forgot. They flavour it with salt. Also they have olives, cheese, and all the veg you need for a real country stew. And for desert they have figs and beans and nuts. And then, after they've supped, they roast acorns and myrtle berries in the fire while they're drinking and chew on them too. They are happy, peaceful and healthy and, when they finally die, their children carry on in the same way.'

Glaucon was always eating sweets and pastries, and we can be pretty sure that he was getting overweight. Plato was concerned about him and by describing a simple happy healthy society he was trying to get across some sound advice about how to go on a diet.

What are we to make of Plato's advice to Glaucon? Of course it is a very old passage, but that does not mean it is out of date. *There is nothing to stop us from following this advice today*! In fact, if we really wanted to, we could follow *exactly* this advice, acorns and all.* But we do not need to go this far. If we go through the foods Plato recommends one by one we can see that we can often safely add a little variety while still keeping within the spirit of the diet.

If you want to try Plato's diet the table tells you what you can eat. You can follow it either as a strict diet, or as an extended diet that uses the same food groups but gives you more choice.

* I am told that acorns make excellent coffee, although as I do not actually drink coffee myself I have never tried it.

Plato's Strict and Extended Diets

STRICT DIET	EXTENDED DIET
wheat and barley	1.all cereals, including unsweetened breakfast cereals 2. rice 3. pasta
bread and [plain] cakes	1. bread 2. (do not kid yourself!), *plain* cakes: no filling, no icing. 3. eggs (a cake ingredient)
wine	wine (*not* 'alcohol!')
salt	1. salt 2. spices
olives	1. plain olives 2. prepared olives
cheese	1.cheese 2. milk 3. plain yoghurt 4. butter
country stew: all vegetables (including potatoes mushrooms, bamboo shoots etc)	all vegetables
figs	all fruit
beans	1. beans 2. beans in sauce, eg baked beans 3. tofu 4. houmous
nuts	all plain or salted nuts
acorns	acorns
myrtle berries	all berries

As you can see from this list, Plato recommends a vegetarian diet, but if you are not a vegetarian, he later talks about eating roast beef and pork and mentions fishing. I think that this means you can reasonably add **meat** and **fish** to the extended diet.

Once non-vegetarians are catered for, you can keep within the spirit of the diet and eat pretty much anything. But if you look through the list, you will find one important exception: you cannot eat sweet tasting food (aside from fruit). If we were to make list of what you could *not* eat, it would start something like this:

* No sugar
* No sugar substitutes
* No honey
* No syrup
* No ice cream
* No chocolate

This list could go on and on and on, but there is no real point in adding to it. You do not need a list like this to know if you are cheating. Imagine that you are tempted by, say, a jam doughnut, and you say to yourself: 'Plato would have approved of me eating this doughnut, because it is basically just a plain cake with some fruit inside—jam is made from fruit—and it's vegetarian too, so if just brush off some of this sugar....' If you find yourself making excuses like this, you know in your heart that you should not eat the thing. And you do not need a big long list of hundreds of banned foods with 'jam doughnuts' as item 127 to tell you not to touch it. What is more, your tongue tells you what is sweet and what's not with perfect accuracy, so as soon as you put something sweet in your mouth, you *know*. In short, there is no need to make a list of banned foods. All we need to remember is one thing:

If it's sweet, don't eat.

What if you eat something sweet by mistake or try something that is sort-of-sweet, or sweeter than you thought it would be? The answer is simple:

If in doubt, spit it out.

Slogans like this are helpful, because they keep things straightforward and easy to remember. With the help of slogans you can keep a diet without needing to look at a list of foods or a chart.

To keep to Plato's diet we need one more slogan:

No more lonely snacks

Lonely snacking is the worst possible thing you can do. Why? Because snacking alone is democratic eating. You are thinking: 'I am free I can do what I like, it is my choice, and other people are nothing to do with it.' So you have a snack. But then you will have another, and then another. That is a sure fire way to get overweight. You are looking to food to satisfy your desire, but your desire for food will never be satisfied, because you will desire more and more and more. In Plato's diet you do the opposite:

(a) you must eat with *ceremony*, and
(b) If possible you must eat with *other people*.

Contrast the fate of the lonely snacker with someone who restricts their eating to regular mealtimes, and does it formally and properly. Of course the meals do not have to be served on plates of reeds while wearing garlands, but you should make an effort of some kind. Wipe the table down; arrange napkins; if you believe in God say grace; light a candle. If you are on your own make a special and deliberate choice of music to listen to. If you are with others, then engage in conversation. When you do this, you think in a different way. The ceremony of eating the food, and (hopefully) the presence of other people, turns eating into an expression of ethical life. This means that you become a part of something bigger, you are making a statement about what you think is right and proper (the formality of preparing the meal), you are using the meal as a way of sharing with others. The food becomes just a part of the atmosphere in the room. The sense of satisfaction you gain is not primarily from the food itself, it is from the ceremony in which it takes place. If you are eating with others a sense of community is gained by sharing with them and talking to them. If you are alone, the candle and the music provide a spiritual community with kindred souls. The kind of satisfaction that this brings does not turn into limitless desire, it brings happiness and a sense of completeness. And because you are thinking in a different way as you eat, you are less likely to eat too much.

What do you do if you *really* want a snack? How do you stop yourself? Plato recommends two things. The first is really simple:

Sing

That's right: *when you feel like a snack, sing a song instead.* It gets you in touch with your spiritual side, so instead of focusing on the greedy desire for food you satisfy your soul. If you can sing with other people, or get them to join in, that will be even better because it will satisfy your need to feel part of a human community.

The second thing you can do instead of having a snack is this:

Get in touch with nature, or more precisely, *sense* nature

Plato suggests going naked or in bare feet outside. The nakedness might be tricky, but going in bare feet is certainly possible. If you have a garden lawn, walk there. Otherwise you can find a park. You are now literally in touch with nature. But of course there are other ways of connecting with nature too, inclulding some that are just as simple and as quick as eating a snack. Here are just a few suggestions.

*Smell a flower
*Climb a tree
* Look at the sky
*If you have time, go a quick walk in the countryside.
*If you are in the middle of the city, walk in the rain *without an umbrella.*
*Take the snack that you would have eaten yourself with you on your walk, and *feed it to an animal instead.*[*]

---

[*] In the countryside there is usually some farm animal that you can feed, and in the town there are almost always pigeons, squirrels, rats etc.

If you can connect with nature and sing at the same time then that will be even better. You will come back feeling good about yourself. And the more you sing and the more you get in touch with nature, the happier you will feel. Snacking is the opposite; the more you snack the more you will feel unhappy.

Glaucon's reply

I had picked up Plato's *Republic* in the original Greek rather than in translation because I did not want Stuart and Wendy to read ahead and see what Glaucon had said about Plato's diet. I had *told* them that Glaucon had been inspired by Plato's description of living off bread, olives, cheese and wine, and had gone on to change his ways, but strictly speaking this was not quite accurate. In fact, I was lying (though only for sound dialectical reasons). What Glaucon had actually said was this:

> 'Yuk Socrates! That diet's only fit for a city of pigs!'
>
> 'Why? What else do they need?'
>
> 'Couches to lie on, tables to eat off and all the delicacies we like today: pastries and nibbles and things.'
>
> 'All right Glaucon. I think our little society is perfectly healthy but if you want one stuffed full with indigestion so be it. I suppose it might help us to learn what's just and what's not. So we'll have it your way and imagine a state with couches and tables, pastries and delicacies, perfume and incense and prostitutes and puddings.'

In other words, Glaucon was rather negative about the diet and refused to try it, and what's more, Plato (in the voice of Socrates) let him off by saying in effect 'OK, we'll see if we can work out another one that allows you to keep all your greedy democratic vices.'

When he eventually found out about this passage, after buying his own translation of *The Republic* in New York, Stuart blamed me for hiding it. He accused me of 'lying' and said that if I had only I told him and Wendy right at the start that Glaucon had said the diet was fit only for pigs, then Wendy might not have gone on the diet at all. This accusation was unfair as Stuart's interpretation was exactly the kind of misreading I wanted to guard against. To the untrained eye many philosophers are difficult if not impossible read at all. Camus for example writes that consciousness 'can only be satisfied by the gratification of its desire. It therefore acts in order to gratify itself and, in so doing, it denies and suppresses its means of gratification.' What does this mean to the average person? Probably nothing.* Plato, however, is easy to read at least at a superficial level, and it is all too easy to imagine that because you can read him you can also understand him. This can make Plato dangerous in the wrong hands.

My First Breakthrough

When I introduced Stuart and Wendy to the diet of pigs I had, to be honest, expected it to fail, but I also thought it would be good for both of them to actually *experience* the diet failing, rather than just rejecting it out of hand. I predicted that Stuart and Wendy's democratic mindset would find the diet too restrictive, because it denied them their right to snack whenever they liked on whatever they liked. The pig diet,

---

* Albert Camus, *The Rebel*, tr. A. Bower (NY: Random House 1956), p. 138. It means (amongst other things) that you eat until you are full, and that as you eat your food disappears, because you have eaten it.

therefore, would not work, but it would give them greater self-knowledge when they tackled the next one.

I was half right because with Stuart this is basically what happened. He had an initial flicker of interest, aroused by the promise that those who follow the diet of pigs have great sex, but he soon succumbed to temptation and eventually I caught him in the bathroom with a packet of doughnuts (he claimed he was brushing the sugar off them). With Wendy, however, something amazing happened. The diet of pigs actually seemed to be working!

I say that this was amazing because I knew that statistically diets almost never work. Of course, I also knew that a philosophical approach to dieting was quite different from the usual 'wonder diet' rubbish, and that in theory at least if you followed a philosopher's advice you could successfully lose weight, but I had not yet realised how astonishingly powerful a philosophical diet could be in practice. It was through Wendy that I learned that if you *linked dieting to a whole way of life*, and if this way of life was something that you responded to eagerly, something that made you grow as a person, then this was the key to losing weight and looking great.

The easiest way of explaining what happened in Wendy's case is to say that the food aspect of the diet was the least important part of the transformation that was taking place before our eyes. Certainly she kept to the rules and never snacked or ate sweet foods. But what was really noticeable was the singing, and the barefoot walks in the park. It was as if these simple things had opened up a new side to life that she had not previously experienced. She would come back to the hotel, her feet splattered in mud, rapturously happy. She would burst in to song repeatedly. It was a tremendous example of a new diet becoming a part of a new life.

'I left my wife in San Francisco'

The singing began to get on Stuart's nerves. He was embarrassed when Wendy sang loudly on the aeroplane as we soared over the Great Plains and the Rockies, and he felt even more awkward when she tried to get him to join in. He opened and shut his mouth like a fish, but no sound came out. He reminded me of myself as a small child pretending to sing hymns in the school assembly.

In San Francisco Wendy began to plait flowers into her hair, and found a bunch of hippies to sing with in the park. She had truly begun to lose weight and look great: the overweight squaw was turning into a flower child. I would glimpse her now and then, seated on the grass surrounded by her new friends. The warm California sunshine, the strumming guitars, the boisterous dogs and laughing scampering children, the handsome bearded young man juggling balls, it all presented an idyllic scene, perhaps not unlike Plato's village. Then, on the last morning before our flight to New York, she was bitten by a squirrel she was feeding and had to have a series of precautionary injections. At this point I still assumed that Wendy's diet was a craze not a profound change. I remember whispering to Stuart in the hospital waiting room that his wife would now quickly lose her enthusiasm for getting close to nature! Stuart, who had long since given up all pretence of keeping to the diet, was frankly relieved. In his childish manner he seemed to think that the squirrel was God's way of making Wendy return to common sense.

We left Wendy in hospital in San Francisco and flew on to New York. Here again, I have been blamed, unfairly, for insisting that we stick to our itinerary. I can only say that if philosophy teaches you anything, it teaches you that you have to take personal responsibility for your own actions. Wendy had been bitten, and that was *her* responsibility. There was no need for us to hang around with her, especially as not only our flight but also our hotel and Broadway tickets had all been pre-booked. By the same token, it was not my fault, although Stuart seemed to think that it was, when instead of flying to meet us in New York, Wendy called to say that she had decided to stay in California and join a commune.

Naturally Stuart was upset about this. That was fair enough. And of course it was unfortunate that they were married. Still it was hard for me to suppress my own excitement at the news. Wendy had been introduced to Plato, she had taken him to heart, and her life had changed. Simply by guiding her, by drawing out and making explicit what Plato was saying about dieting, I had been the midwife of that change. Here, already, was real concrete evidence of what a philosophical approach to dieting could do. I was elated, I felt like a child when they first learn to ride a bicycle. I had done it! It was my first real success and, for all that happened later, one that still fills me with quiet pride.

Stuart insisted on flying back to the West Coast to try and locate his wife. He was an adult and it was his choice. For myself, it was with a vastly increased confidence in the philosophy of dieting that I returned, alone, to the UK to continue my sessions with the other Guinea Pigs. But I was also cautious. Philosophical dieting was obviously very potent and needed to be handled carefully to avoid unintended consequences. All in all, after what happened with Stuart and

Wendy I decided to not to introduce the diet of pigs to the other Guinea Pigs, and warned them against reading *The Republic*. Instead I moved on to another and—as I thought—safer philosopher: Thomas Hobbes.

The Diet of Pigs in a Nutshell

1. If it's sweet, don't eat.
2. If in doubt, spit it out.
3. No snacks.
4. Sense nature.
5. Sing.

Sources

Plato, *The Republic*
GWF Hegel, *Philosophy of Right*

Dear Edna
I am back from holiday so this is just to let you know that the philosophy of dieting sessions will be starting again in the church hall. There will be four of us. (No need to make us anything of course!)
Very Best Wishes,
Peter

PS The bagels in New York are fantastic, but your homemade buns are <u>even better</u>.

Chapter 3
Hobbes's Diet Contract

which explains how once you have promised to go on a diet, you can be made to stick to that promise.

Do not break the law. Follow the rules. How we are drilled into this. How shameful to appear in court charged with some offence! Yet when it comes to dieting rules, we break them all the time. The diet contract is based on a simple idea: we try and extend our attitude to the law to diets. In the diet contract you treat breaking your diet as seriously as any other form of law breaking: as criminal. The hoped for result is that you will no more think of becoming a diet-criminal than you would of committing any other violation of the law. This is the dieting philosophy explained by Thomas Hobbes.

There was something rather odd about Hobbes. While other children laughed and played he would sit in the corner reading Greek. While other teenagers lay in bed in the mornings, the youthful Hobbes would get up early to amuse himself by killing jackdaws. And if he *did* stay in bed, he would get out his pen, ruler and compass to draw geometrical shapes on the flesh of his own thighs. Later, as a young adult Hobbes was known for his unhealthy features. His feet were always damp and he had yellow skin—not a glorious oriental hue, but a bilious colour that made him appear permanently unwell. Although the chroniclers are not explicit, I think that we can safely assume that this 'ill looking' man was also significantly overweight. And herein lies the mystery of Thomas Hobbes.

When Hobbes reached the age of 40, suddenly everything changed. People began to remark how great he looked, how his appearance had altered for the better. He cheered up. His hair glistened black. He was bursting with health, his face gained 'a fresh, ruddy complexion.' Hobbes went on to live to 91, a ripe old age even today and almost unheard of back in the seventeenth century. Furthermore, this was no clinging on. He went hiking and swimming. He sang—especially in bed, and he was also, in the strictest sense of the term, a bit of a love machine, with a succession of girlfriends. The last of these, the beautiful Mary Dell, had an intimate relationship with him in the very year of his death. How could this be? The answer is that Hobbes had worked out the secret to losing weight and looking great. I say 'secret' because he never set down exactly how he did it. To be sure there are some nuggets of practical advice scattered about here and there: have regular meals, do not scoff lots of food even if it is fruit in season; eat fish in preference to meat. What is apparently lacking is a whole dieting philosophy. But it is there all right; it lies just below the surface in his main philosophical works.

The Basic Diet Contract

Thomas Hobbes described life as 'solitary, poor, nasty, brutish and short'. But Hobbes wasn't talking about *all* life, only life in what he called 'the state of nature.' So what did Hobbes mean by this? Well, he once described the state of nature as being like a Native American living in the woods, but this can be a bit misleading, because the 'nature' is actually nothing to do with trees and rivers and things like that, it is to do with *freedom.* Native Americans were free because in the state of nature, *there isn't any law.* This means that it is a state in which you can do *whatever you like.* You can do absolutely anything, from your wildest dreams to your most repulsive fantasies. Because there is no law, there is *nothing* to stop you, you can just *go for it* because you are *totally* unconstrained.

I want you to stop and just think for a minute what you might do, living in a state of nature. What *urges* or *desires* would you have? *How* would you fulfil them? Make a mental list of three things, or, better, write them down.

In the state of nature, this is what I would do:

1.____

2.____

3.____

When you have had enough day dreaming you can answer this question too:

Q. What did Hobbes say we would do in the state of nature?

A.____

I wonder if you got the right answer? Hobbes said that *we would all go around killing each other.*

Hobbes does not have a very optimistic view of humanity. He thinks that we are fundamentally selfish as (1) we are greedy, (2) we lie and (3) we really enjoy feeling more important than everyone else. This means that given the chance we would kill each other, sometimes in order to steal, sometimes because we did not trust each other, and sometimes just to sort of show off that we could. Hobbes has a solution to this. To get out of the dreadful state of nature we must choose someone—anyone—to be in charge of making the law, and then everyone else must promise to obey that law.

In the seventeenth century this argument was new. Plenty of other people had said you should obey the law, but they had explained this by arguing: (1) The law comes from the King and (2) the King has been chosen by God. Therefore, (3) the law comes from God. Thanks to Hobbes, we do not believe that any longer. But in a way we still do. All of the glitter and glitz around a king, prime minister, or president makes them celebrities, and that makes it easy to think that they are somehow a very special kind of person. Really, they are not. They are just ordinary, like you. They might be quite good at pretending that they are not ordinary, but underneath, they are, and some of them are very ordinary indeed. Once you realise that your President—or whoever—is really very ordinary your disillusionment can actually be quite dangerous, because you may then think: 'Why listen to *them*. Who are *they* to boss us around? Why obey the law?' That is when revolutions start and people start getting their heads cut off.

Hobbes gave us a new reason to do as we are told and a very good one, because it applies even if our lawmakers are arrogant, dim witted, mean spirited and generally rather contemptible.

'Yes,' argued Hobbes, 'our sovereigns are ordinary' ('sovereign' was Hobbes's preferred word for the leader of a country). 'And No, the sovereigns *don't* have a special relationship with God or anything else that makes them better than the rest us. But we must still obey the law.' Why? 'It is as if we are standing on the edge of a precipice, all of us, and once we start breaking the law, we will slip off and fall into a state of nature. And that is going to be nasty.' We can add that in all probability it will be *very* nasty, and it will certainly be far worse than being bossed around a bit by a sovereign.

This argument made Hobbes famous. But there is something implicit in it that has escaped notice. In a state of nature, people do not *just* go round killing each other. They *also* go around eating too much (mainly because they are greedy).

Have a look back at your list of what you would do in a state of nature. Now, I sincerely hope that your list does not include things like 'kill my neighbour and eat everything in his fridge.' I hope it says nicer things than that, and *I* am sure that you are telling the *truth*. But Hobbes is a bit of a cynic, and so if you say that you would do nice things, *Hobbes* simply thinks that you are *lying* and that you would actually be every bit as nasty and greedy as everyone else.

Hobbes's state of nature is not that different from what Plato's democracy. There is the same logic in each case: you can do whatever you like—so you overeat. And all the five classic results of being overweight follow, from being lonely (solitary), to having a reduced life expectancy (short). But with Hobbes we also get a very different and very ingenious solution to this problem.

Remember how Glaucon told Socrates: 'I'm not going on a pig's diet!'? Glaucon's problem was that although the diet of pigs was a sensible one, it did not fit in with his 'prostitutes and puddings' lifestyle. Hobbes understands this type of problem. He realises that a diet that makes you change your whole life is unlikely to work. So he goes for realism, creating a form of diet that people can easily follow because it *fits in with their daily lives.* Of course, people's lives in the seventeenth century were not exactly like ours, but with fantastic foresight Hobbes's diet not only worked back then, but still works today. In fact it probably works *better* now than it has ever done in the past.

Hobbes's brilliant innovation was to invent the diet *contract*. We all know about contracts because they an integral part of everyday life. You make a contract to get an internet connection, use a mobile phone, go on holiday, hire a car. Tenancy agreements, mortgages and bank loans, and terms of employment are all forms of contract. The diet contract is nothing out of the ordinary, it's just one more piece of paper to sign. Compare this with the diet of pigs and you can immediately see the advantage. In the pig diet you had to make an effort to stand back from mainstream society, if not drop out altogether and be a 'hippy.' The diet contract *is* mainstream: you are making contracts all the time, why not make another one? And it is a particularly easy contract to enter into, because, if you want to lose weight then why not? Even better, there is no chance of being cheated into signing up for something you do not really want to do; Hobbes's idea is to base the contract on your own wishes and your own self-knowledge. This means that the person who draws up the terms of the contract is *you.*

I have made a couple of templates for you to choose from. One is a 'classic' contract, the other a 'modern' contract. You can use whichever you are most comfortable with, but in either case, it is *your* job to fill in the blanks. The words in the classic contract are a bit old-fashioned, as though Hobbes might have written them. The modern contract says the same thing in today's terms.

The Classic Contract

I, ___________________ being of sound mind but of corpulent body, do earnestly declare that I intend to lose weight. Pursuant to this declared intention I do, furthermore, hereby make a most solemn covenant to henceforth observe the following dieting rules:

Rule 1____

Rule 2____

The above stated dieting rules will be come into effect immediately forthwith in their full rigor. They apply on all days of the year, with the exception of the following special occasions for indulging in excess:

Excessive Occasion 1____

Excessive Occasion 2____

On all other days, I do most faithfully swear to uphold the dieting rules until the moment of my death or until the following date, whichever be the sooner:

End of Contract Date____________________

Any deviation or breach of the rules on any date other than those expressly appointed for the indulgement of excess will incur, immediately, the following penalty.

Penalty for Breach of Rule

____

The above penalty I do most heartily agree to undergo were I to transgress on my promise in any way, confident as I am that in my settled resolve to lose weight the stricture is entirely otiose and wholly superfluous.

All that is set down hereunto in the aforesaid do I vow to follow, in affirmation whereof I do hereby sign my name in the presence of the hereafter stated witnesses thereof.

Signed ____________________________

Witness 1 (name and signature)

____

Witness 2 (name and signature)

____

Date________________________

The Modern Contract

I, ____________________ admit it. I'm fat. I need to lose weight. To do that I promise I will follow these rules:

Rule

1____

Rule

2____

I will always follow these rules, apart from occasional times when I can forget about them. These times are:

Forget the rules time 1

____

Forget the rules time 2

____

I will follow the rules, either until I am dead, or until the final day of this contract which is:

End of Contract Date_____________________

Whenever I break the rules (at times when I am not allowed to) this will happen:

Penalty for Breach of Rule

____

Will I really do that? Yes. But to be honest, the penalty doesn't matter, because I want to lose weight so much that there is no way I am going to break the rules in the first place.

I promise to do all of this stuff in front of two witnesses who have signed their names below mine.

Signed __________________________

Witness 1 (name and signature)

____

Witness 2 (name and signature)

____

Date________________________

That's the contract, now we need to work out how you are going to fill it in, beginning with the rules.

Rules

Go for things that are simple, doable and unambiguous. Here are some examples: no cheese; no food after 8pm; no second-helpings.

Special Occasions for Excess/Forgetting the Rules

Hobbes had a special occasion about every nine months, so once or twice a year is about right. Try and specify dates or time periods eg 'Christmas 24 Dec-1 Jan' inclusive or 'Summer Holiday (2 weeks maximum).'

End Date

If you do not want to tie yourself in for the rest of your life, put an end date in. If it has worked in the meantime, you can then make another one. I suggest one year.

Penalties

Hobbes seems to have had two penalties. First, he would play a game of tennis *even though he didn't like it.* This is an excellent example of a penalty. Indeed, *provided* that you do not like tennis, or find it inconvenient and expensive to organise, then writing in 'play a game of tennis' under the penalty clause of your contract works every bit as well today. I thoroughly recommend it.

Thomas Hobbes playing tennis

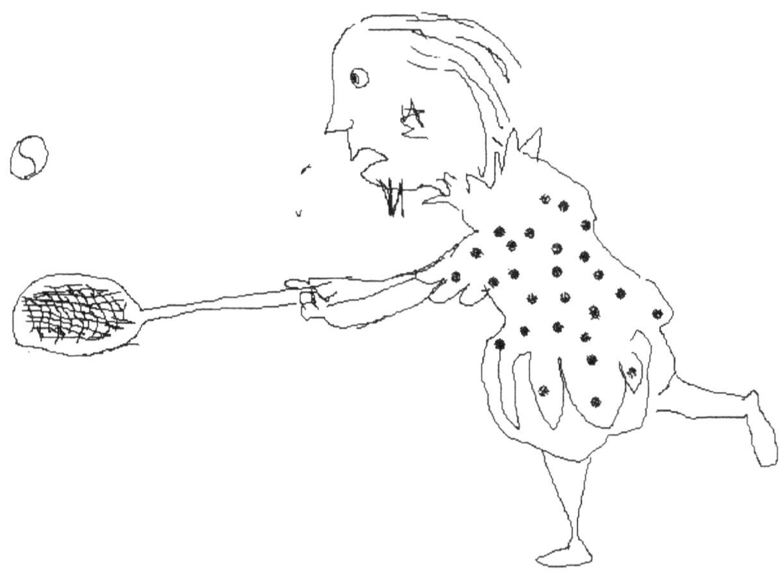

Observe the general principle behind the tennis penalty; you want to identify a vigorous physical activity that you do *not* find enjoyable. It can be outdoorsy or sporting, and it can also be useful. However, you must be careful not to incur as a penalty things that you need to do *anyway*. For example, 'Mow the lawn' is suspect as a penalty, because every time the grass needs cutting, you will be tempted to break your diet and pig-out, and instead of a penalty, you will get a reward of food for what you should do in any event. By contrast, if you have as a penalty: 'Mow my *neighbour's* lawn,' that would be excellent because it is a physically demanding chore that you would not otherwise do. And if you happen to dislike your neighbour, so much the better.

Hobbes imposed a second penalty upon himself too. And here I have to be careful, because I am stuck between two things. (1) I want to tell *the truth*. No matter what it is, no matter how dark, ugly, unpalatable, un-pc. That is what philosophy is all about, the love of truth. (2) I don't want to break the law in any way, or get sued.

So let's get the legal issue out of the way. Please read the following warning very carefully.

WARNING

HOBBES'S SECOND DIET PENALTY IS NOT RECOMMENDED. IN FACT, YOU ARE STRONGLY ADVISED *NOT* TO DO IT.

IF YOU DISREGARD THIS ADVICE YOUR TEETH (without expensive cosmetic dentistry) WILL TURN *PERMANENTLY* YELLOW.

AND YOUR BREATH WILL SMELL.

Got that? OK. Not to put too fine a point on it, Hobbes's second penalty for breaking his diet was simply to put two fingers down his throat to make himself vomit. He would do this so often that it actually became a bit of a 'party trick,' so that he was celebrated for his ability to be sick *while simultaneously carrying on a conversation*. In fact, it was said that he found it so easy to make himself sick that 'neither his wit was disturbed (longer than he was spewing) nor his stomach oppressed.' Now, the brutal philosophical truth about this penalty is that it works. It is an effective deterrent: swift, sure and immediate self-retribution, and if you do break the rules and eat more than you should, then the food is voided before you have time to digest it. For proof of its efficacy , one only has to look at images of Princess Diana, who often made herself sick and who looked not just great but *fabulous.* But still, I want to repeat my earnest advice not to do this yourself. It is rather like a circus stunt: *they* can do it, but *you* should not. There is—emphatically—NO GUARANTEE that you will end up looking as beautiful as Princess Di. And, as I have already intimated, all that stomach acid will do your teeth no good at all.

The Sovereign Partner Diet

At our meeting in the church hall I explained Hobbes's philosophy of dieting to the three remaining Guinea Pigs, Angie, Jasmine and Derek, and handed out contracts. They were enthusiastic and, after we had had eaten the Vicars wife's cream scones, everyone filled one in with their own rules and penalties. Angie said her rule was no snacks and that as a penalty she would go running before breakfast. Jasmine's rule was no second helpings; she did not say what her penalty was to be. Derek also promised not to snack and, taking things too far, promised to cut a finger off every time he broke his diet.

A week later we sat down with our tea and cake in the church hall to compare notes. Jasmine looked like she might have lost a bit of weight, but she was coy about whether she had kept to the rules. Angie had broken her rule twice already, and been up and running. The thing was, she said, she had found that she actually rather *enjoyed* her run. This problem was simple to solve by making a minor adjustment to her contract. Angie had been setting off for her runs at seven in the morning. In future, when she broke her diet she was to set off at *two* in the morning. Derek's dilemma was more complicated. All of his fingers were intact, and the reason was simple: he had been cheating. Just as Hobbes predicted, human beings are often greedy and deceitful so they will, naturally enough, break their promise and then, instead of taking their punishment, say 'Whoops. Oh well. I forgive myself.'

At this point there was a knock at the door. I assumed it was Edna with seconds so I was most surprised when Stuart entered. The last time I had seen Stuart, in New York, he had been brandishing his translation of Plato's *Republic* and accusing me of ruining his marriage. But I am not one to bear grudges, and welcomed him back. Jasmine sorted out his tea and cakes and Angie asked gently about Wendy. Stuart had apparently spoken to her at the commune and that they had struck a deal. Wendy *would* come back, but only *after* he had lost weight. So that was why he was here. What was the next diet? He was willing to try anything, *anything*. Except the pig diet again; that had not worked for him. It was not the food so much, it was the bare feet: his feet were sensitive. But any other diet, even the most *extreme*, he was up for it.

There was a great deal of sympathy for Stuart, the girls fussed over him like mother hens and even Derek was kind to him in a tom cat sort of way.

'Don't sit on your own every night Stu,' he said 'That's a sure way to eat too much. Get out on the town with me instead.'

'Thanks Derek. I'd like that. It's a bit lonely in that big house without Wendy.'

'Yeah, unhealthy too. You come with us and we'll have a good *prowl around*.'

I was glad Stuart had turned up when he did because it opened up the possibility of trying a further variation on the diet contract. I told him about it and he was keen to join in. Then, I posed a problem. Stuart might *say* that he promised to follow the diet contract, but he'd said the same the last time. I did not want Stuart to think I was prejudiced, against him. But when all was said and done, when we had tried the pig diet I *had* found him in the bathroom with a packet of donuts. So if Stuart broke the rules again how was the penalty to be paid?

Brows furrowed, the Guinea Pigs sat in thought.

It was Angie who worked out the answer, at least in principle.

'We need *you* to be Stuart's sovereign!' she exclaimed.

Everyone gasped. The solution was so obvious, so simple: a sovereign to enforce the rules.

'Of course! exclaimed Stuart 'When I break my diet, you can punish me!'

'Perhaps you can be a sovereign for all of us' continued Angie, 'We can come here every week, and if we've broken the rules, you can, um…'

There was another pause.

'Yes, your line of thinking is spot on.' I said. 'Keep on going. Perhaps think back to how things were in the old days when things were simpler.'

'You can do things like whip us,' suggested Jasmine shyly.

The idea that the Guinea Pigs needed a sovereign with the power to punish them was completely sound 'Covenants without the sword are but words' Hobbes had said. By this he meant that making a promise (a 'covenant') on its own is no good without a punishment (a 'sword') for those who break them. So the logic of what was being suggested was impeccable and it probably would have worked. But even though it appeared entirely above board, I vaguely sensed that there could be some kind of legal comeback were I to start whipping Guinea Pigs. Philosophy can only be taken so far, one must also obey the laws of the state. Indeed it was on this very point that Hobbes was so insistent.

So I knocked it on the head.

'Whoa there GPs!' I said. (I had started to call the Guinea Pigs 'GPs' as a collective nickname.) 'I'm here to be your friend, your mentor, your kindly uncle, your shoulder to cry on. But I'm not here to be your sovereign. Let's get back to sorting one out for Stuart. It's a great idea to have a sovereign. But can I ask one of *you* to volunteer?

There was a silence.

'Please guys,' said Stuart, 'I really want to get back with Wendy.'

There was another silence. Finally Angie spoke.

'I'll do it.'

'Thanks Angie I appreciate it,' said Stuart feelingly.

I appreciated it too. Angie was a very caring person, and I liked her more and more.

We had a little ceremony where Stuart formally pledged to obey Angie as his sovereign, and then I explained about the type of diet they were entering into: *the sovereign partner diet*.

Anyone can be your sovereign. Hobbes is quite explicit that it doesn't matter who it is, as long as you have one. So for the sovereign partner diet a friend will do as a sovereign, or even someone you do not like very much. However, it if you are married it is best, if possible, to get your spouse to act as sovereign. Marriage is meant to be about love, but when you say 'I do' you are actually making a contract, and one with real and powerful legal implications. When you break a marriage law, your spouse is like your sovereign king or queen: they are the person whose law you have broken. Once that is realised, it is a simple matter to add dieting laws to the marriage vows.

Marriage is a special type of contract because when you get married you promise to *forgo* things, to do without certain pleasures. Marriage, therefore, is a *diet.* In fact, it's a contract to go on a diet. You must not be unfaithful, but that is no excuse to gain weight instead. Indeed, at a philosophical level, it could be argued that having an 'affair' with a large packet of crisps is not that different from having an affair with a colleague.

I am not, of course, saying that your spouse should divorce you if you become overweight. What I am saying is that a spouse (or partner) can help you diet by enforcing the penalties. For husbands and wives, or anyone in a live-in relationship, there is a natural penalty: if you break the diet, you do the domestic chores usually done by the *other* partner. If, for example, they usually do the vacuuming, then if you break your diet *you* have to do it.

This modifies the basic contract a bit. You can cut out the witnesses and put your partner's name there instead—like this in the modern contract:

Modern Contract with Sovereign Partner

I, ____________________ admit it. I'm fat. I need to lose weight. To do that I promise I will follow these rules:

Rule

1____

Rule

2____

I will always follow these rules, apart from occasional times when I can forget about them. These times are:

Forget the rules time

1____

Forget the rules time

2____

I will follow the rules, either until I am dead, or until the final day of this contract which is:

End of Contract Date_____________________

Whenever I break the rules this will happen:

Penalty for Breach of Rule

____

Will I really do that? Yes. Because my partner will make me.

Signed __________________________

Partner
(signature)_________________________________

Date________________________

In short, the advantage of having a sovereign partner is they can interfere with you and boss you around to keep you on your diet.

Two Phone Calls

Stuart and Angie filled out the contract together. They worked out a simple rule: no food from 8pm until breakfast. What was the penalty to be? Angie suggested that she make Stuart go on a three mile run. Stuart shook his head:

'Not painful enough,' he said dismissively, 'and anyway I haven't got a tracksuit.'

I left them to sort out the details.

In the following week I was surprised to receive two 'real' phone calls on the same day. I should explain that after my wife left me I had led an essentially solitary existence. I call her my wife, but we were not really together for all that long. I met her over the internet at the time I was writing the script about the orphan girl with Knudson, and indeed it was at Knudson's suggestion that I should say that I was an international film maker rather than an academic when I advertised myself to prospective brides from abroad. So I did, the trick worked, and at first things went well, but after the film fell through my wife walked out. Her parting shot, 'I thought I marry a film maker and I find I marry a fat professor from the university of nowhere,' had hurt. After that, I retreated from life. Like a wounded animal hiding beneath a bush I had stayed away from the social whirl and immersed myself in my philosophical work. It was very unusual, therefore, to receive these two 'proper' phone calls.

The first call was from Angie, who sounded anxious.

'Peter, I've got a problem,' she said. 'I broke my diet rule again, so I went a run through the town at two in the morning.'

Good. Well done Angie. That sounds more like you've *solved* a problem. Was the run unpleasant?'

'Not very nice no.'

'Great!'

'I thought I'd stay in the town because I felt safer there.'

'Yes, sensible. But with all those bars and "gentlemen's clubs", it must be pretty disgusting at that time?'

'Yes, it is: full of drunks and vomit. The thing is though, when I went across the bridge I saw Stuart, and he was breaking his diet.'

'Stuart? Are you sure?'

'I saw him eating. Stuart and Derek were both there, eating chips and kebabs.'

'But Stuart isn't meant to eat from 8 pm until breakfast time!'

'Exactly. I mean, what should I do now?'

'Perhaps it wasn't really him? It must have been dark.'

'It was Stuart all right. He hid his face in his chips, but it was Stuart I'm sure of it.'

'Then I don't see any problem Angie', I said firmly. 'Stuart has made a contract. He has been caught red handed breaking it. Confront him at our next meeting, secure his confession and impose the penalty.'

'Yes I know that's the theory, but I didn't really think last week when we drew it up that I would actually have too *do* it. I mean, couldn't I just pretend that I didn't see him?'

'Angie, Stuart *knows* you've seen him, otherwise why would he have tried to hide his face? And you're not just friends any longer, you're his sovereign. If this diet is going to work, if he's going to get Wendy back, he's *got* to follow the contract.'

Angie sighed. 'OK, I'll see if I can borrow one.'

The second call was from Wendy. It was a poor line and the constant noise of throbbing pop music, barking dogs and crying babies made it even more difficult to hear. But it went something like this.

'Peter?'

(Woomp! Woof! Waa!)

'What?'

Peter it's Wendy!'

(Woomp! Woof! Waa!)

'Wendy how nice to hear from you!'

'Yes.'

'Guess what Wendy, you're the second girl to phone me up today!'

(Woomp! Woof! Waa!)

'Am I?'

'Are you having a nice time in the commune?'

(Woomp! Woof! Waa!)

'Yes, yes it's great.'

'Quite different from living in a house in a village in the middle of the English countryside. I expect!'

(Woomp! Woof! Waa!)

'Pardon?'

'Must-Be-Different?'

'Yes.'

'But fun I'm sure. I've always wondered Wendy, are the bedrooms…'

'What? Anyway Peter. I'm calling about Stuart.'

'Yes?'

'Is he coming to the meetings?'

'Yes!'

'Good. And is he trying to diet?'

'Well, I mean...'

Given what I had just heard from Angie, this was a tricky question to answer. However, before I had decided whether to reply truthfully or dialectically our conversation was interrupted. For in the background, rising above the noises of the music, animals and children I could hear the call of an insistent male voice.

'Wendy! Oh Wendy!'

'Hold on a minute Jester.'

'What?'

'Nothing: it's just someone at my end. I mean, I'm thinking it's silly, if he's really trying to diet, to ...'

'Tantric yoga time Wendy!'

'Oh Gawd. Jester, let go!'

Then the phone went dead.

It was difficult to know what to make of this phone call. Certainly there was no mention from Wendy that she was going to fly straight back, so that I can hardly be blamed that she turned up at an inconvenient moment. But the fact of the matter was that she did, and then, when she found that the church hall door was locked, had gone next door to the Vicar, which made things worse. But I am jumping ahead of myself. Before we get to what happened, we need to bring in another philosopher.

Descartes' Mind Body Diet

From what Angie had told me, Derek too had obviously been breaking his diet. So before the next meeting I had to devise a strategy for him.

To solve the problem of cheats like Derek I looked to the philosopher, René Descartes. Descartes had a simple idea: we have a body and we have a mind, and they are separate. Christians believe this—or at least something similar—when they separate our mortal body from our immortal soul. But even atheists can concede that there is a physiological justification for the mind body distinction, because as well as the brain in our head, we have a second much more primitive type of brain in our stomach, loosely akin to the nervous system of a jellyfish. So whichever way you look at it, religious or not, we are not really one person but two. And like any two people we quarrel. In fact, there is a recurring argument going on inside use between our mind and our body. In this argument, it is the body that is demanding too much food. The mind, rationally, merely wants to give the body enough. The body, however, is not satisfied with enough. It nags for more than it should get, and when the mind is weak, it sometimes gives in.

To make this clear to the GPs I quickly sketched a couple of diagrams on the whiteboard of the church hall. The first diagram ('Cartesian Dualism') shows that what we do is not the decision of one person, but the result of a fight between two people—the mind and the body. The second diagram ('Fluctuating Will') presents three graphs to show how both our mind *and* our body have a will that changes in strength. If the will of our mind is consistently stronger than our body, we stay slim. If our body always has a stronger will than our mind, we get overweight. But if the will of each fluctuates up and down enough then sometimes the will of the mind is stronger than the body, and sometimes the will of the body is stronger than the mind. The result is that our weight goes up and down. This is typical for a person on a diet: they diet when the will of the mind is in a strong fluctuation and the will of the body is weak, and break the diet when the will of the body becomes strong and the mind weakens. Then as the mind strengthens, and body weakens, they return to dieting, and so on.

Cartesian Dualism

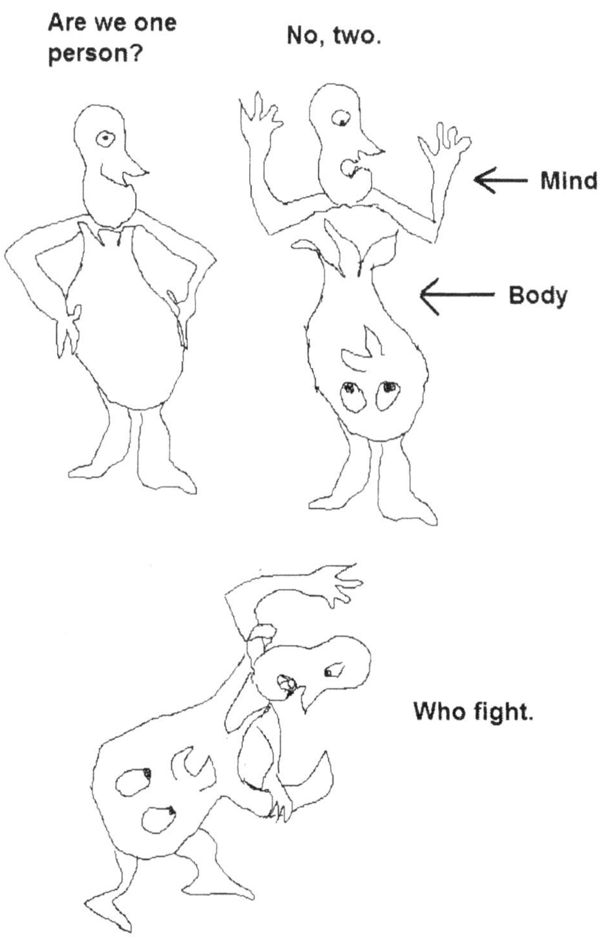

Fluctuating Will

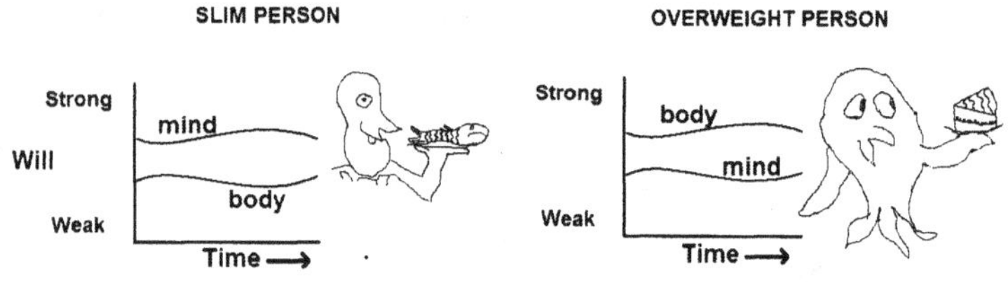

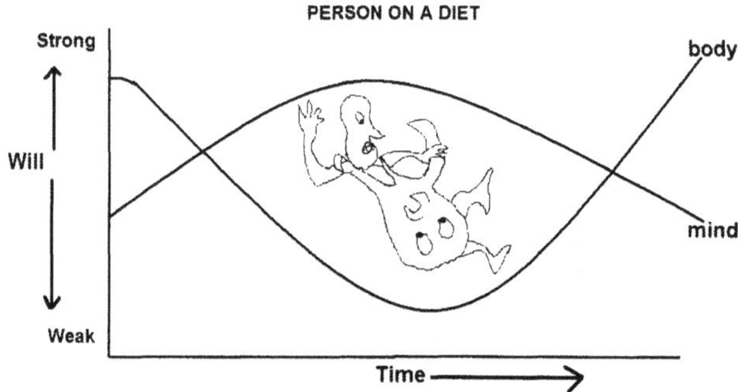

We can combine Descartes insight that there are two of us with Hobbes's idea of writing something down, making a formal statement. But this time we are not going to put it in the form of a contract, rather we will write a letter—to ourselves. More specifically, we are going to write a letter from our mind *when it is strong*, to our mind *when it is weak*.

Imagine you have just eaten a huge packet of crisps. Your body is happy, your mind is distraught.

'Oh No!' exclaims your mind. 'Why did I do that? Why did I listen to my greedy body?'

'Sucker,' gurgles your body and dozes off.

Now, when it seems too late, your mind is clear and strong. But is it too late? No! Because now is the time to communicate with your mind in the future, when you reach for the *next* bag of crisps. Seize the moment. Grab pen and paper and write. Pour out your heart about how revolting it is to eat too much, about how it makes you overweight and unhappy. As soon as you are done, seal the letter in an envelope, address it to yourself, and put it somewhere, where you will find it when next tempted to break your diet. Promise to yourself that when this happens, before you break your diet you will do one thing. You will read this letter *and answer it.*

Another diagram, 'Corresponding with yourself', shows this: When your mind is strong and your body weak, you write the letter, when your body is strong and your mind is weak, you read the letter. When that moment of weakness comes, your body will know that this letter is fatal to its plans. It will say: 'don't open that letter.' Because it knows if you do, you can't answer it: it is impossible to answer.

Corresponding with yourself

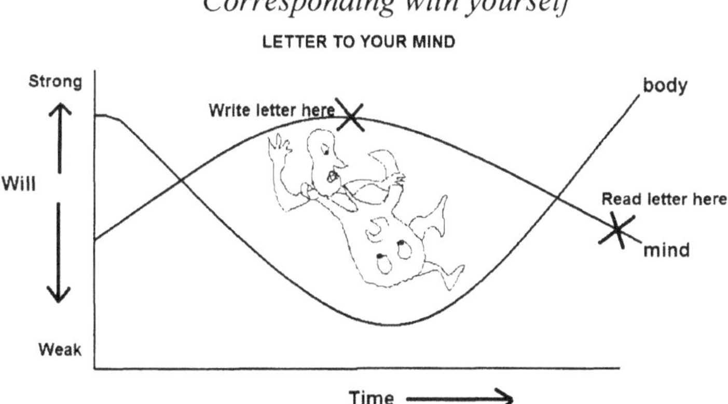

Incident with the Vicar

At our next meeting I explained Descartes' diet to Derek, Stuart and Angie. We now had two types of diet to follow, so we split into two groups. I went into the kitchen with Derek to help him with the mind body diet, while Stuart and Angie stayed in the main hall to continue the sovereign partner diet.

The pretence that Knudson and the A Team were on a tropical island somewhere continued to be a useful spur to get the GPs to diet, so I had thus far delayed telling them the truth. For this reason I was, fortunately, still filming the so-called 'TV documentary.' I say fortunately, because it meant that I had a record of what happened and was able to play it to the police, although of course it should never have got that far. The problem was that there were two copies of the key, and if anything, as we had booked the venue, they should have arrested the Vicar for trespassing, rather than wasting public money following up an idiotic complaint about what two perfectly respectable people were doing in the privacy of their own local church hall.

I provide the relevant part of the transcript from the film below, so that you can judge for yourselves. The camcorder was on in the small kitchen area in the back but it was the 'noises off' in the main hall that caused all the fuss. Jasmine has insisted on my adding that she had nothing to do with it. Indeed, she was not in attendance that week because she happened to have been hospitalised for bulimia.

TRANSCRIPT 2

INT. DAY. CHURCH HALL, KITCHEN

PETER: (to camera) While Stuart prepares to be punished by his 'sovereign' Angie in the main hall, Derek and I retreated to the kitchen to start working on another document. It's a letter.

DEREK: (speaks as he writes) 'Dear Derek'...Now what?

PETER: You were telling me that after you've eaten a packet of crisps, you feel really disgusted with yourself?

DEREK: Yes, I do.

PETER: Great! Now write those feelings down.

PETER: (to camera) Derek has not got a partner or trusted friend at the moment, so unlike Stuart he can't make a contract that will be enforced by someone else. In a sense, what Derek is going to do is to make a contract with himself in the letter he's writing. Now you might think that this is impossible because a contract requires at least two people. And Hobbes would probably agree; it *is* impossible. So that's why we're going to borrow an idea from another great philosopher and a contemporary of Hobbes, René Descartes.

DEREK: (reading out) 'You will kid yourself that you are only going to eat one. But you won't. Once you eat one crisp, you'll scoff the whole lot, the whole blooming packet will go down your big gullet.'

PETER: Good. Now add all those feelings you'll have once you've eaten them.

PETER: (to camera) Descartes had a simple idea: we are made up of two things, a mind and a body. It's the body that demands that we eat, and if the mind doesn't stop it, it just keeps on demanding, until we eat too much.

DEREK: (reading out) 'After you've eaten those crisps, you will feel like a loathsome little slug.'

PETER (Prompts): 'Little'? Don't you mean 'fat'?

DEREK. (crossing out and rewriting) 'You will feel like a loathsome fat slug. You will feel worthless, like it would be best if someone could just come along and tread on you, like a slug.'

PETER: That's a bit hard on slugs isn't it? ...

NOISES OFF
ANGIE: One! [Crack]
STUART Aagh!

PETER: (to camera) To understand what Derek is doing, we can put Descartes' idea another way. Derek is compulsive eater. Compulsive eaters are not one person. They are *two* people. The first person is ruled by the body and who loves compulsive eating. The second person is ruled by the mind and hates compulsive eating.

DEREK: (reading out) 'You will feel bloated, sick, smelly...'

NOISES OFF
ANGIE: Two! [Crack]
STUART Aagh!

DEREK: [Chews pencil, frowns and continues to write]

PETER: (to camera) So what Derek is doing is writing a letter when his mind, which hates compulsive eating, is in control, to a time when his body, which loves it, takes over

DEREK: (reading out) 'Yours sincerely, Derek.'

NOISES OFF
ANGIE: Three! [Crack]
STUART Aagh!

DEREK: [Signs letter with flourish and reads it through with look of stern resolution]

PETER: (to camera) When Derek has his next craving for crisps, he's promised himself just one thing. He can eat the crisps, eat as many as he likes. But there's something he's go to do first. Read and answer that letter.

PETER: Great Derek. Now let's find an envelope and you can stick it on the cupboard, when you get home.

NOISES OFF
ANGIE: Four! [Crack]
STUART Aagh!
Door Opens
VICAR: What on earth is going on?
WENDY: Stuart!
STUART: Darling!

PETER AND DEREK: [Ears perk up, exchange of puzzled glances]

NOISES OFF

ANGIE: Oh hello Wendy! Vicar. It's a bit odd I know but it's just our regular dieting meeting.

VICAR: What?

ANGIE I didn't realise you were back Wendy. Do you want to take over?

WENDY; Oh Stuart! what have they done to you?

ANGIE: I've just got a few more to go. Ow! Stop it! Wendy! Ouch!

VICAR I'll call the police!

PETER: Hold on Derek (reaches for camera). I'd better just...

SCREEN GOES BLANK

By this point I had obviously become aware that the main session in the hall had been interrupted, and went in to 'pour oil on troubled waters.' Derek followed, and together with Stuart we managed to restrain Wendy before she caused too much injury to Angie. I explained what was going on and how it was all perfectly normal and would help Stuart to lose weight. Stuart explained that it hadn't hurt as much as it sounded and that Angela had actually been quite gentle, certainly much gentler than Wendy, and eventually Wendy calmed down.

The Vicar however—and this is typical of the fraught relationship between philosophy and religion—was less forgiving. I will not set down our conversation, as there is little to be gained from becoming embroiled in argument with an excitable indignant man, hot under the dog collar, with no understanding of the philosophical significance of what we were doing. But I think the excerpt is enough to vindicate me, and of course this was the police's view, else why would they have decided not to prosecute? The Vicar then tried to ban us from the church hall. But this I refused to accept, pointing out that we had booked and paid for the hall in advance and any attempt to exclude us would invoke the full weight of the law for a breach of contract. So the Vicar had to be content with saying that his wife was not going to provide us with any more cakes, to which I said that this was up to *her*, not *him*. I only wish to add that Derek's later insinuation that I had somehow encouraged or even instigated the whole thing is utterly scurrilous.

The Diet Contract in a Nutshell

1. The Basic Contract:
Set dieting rules, allow yourself a couple of exceptions and identify penalties involving some form of physical exercise.
2. The Sovereign Partner Diet
Get your partner to enforce the penalties.
3. The Mind Body Diet
Write a letter to yourself and promise yourself to read and answer it before breaking your diet.

Sources

J. Aubrey, *Brief Lives*
R. Descartes, *Meditations*
GWF Hegel, *Philosophy of Right*
T. Hobbes, *Leviathan*
T. Hobbes, *De Cive*
T. Hobbes, *De Mirabilibus Pecci*
T. Hobbes, *The Life of Mr. Thomas Hobbes of Malmesbury*
T. Hobbes, letter to Aubrey, 30 June 1664

Dear Edna,
I am SO sorry about what happened. Of course your husband was upset. He had every right to be. And I am not going to defend myself, No. All I am going to do is say thank you. Because your food has been so delicious, so wonderful! The teacakes, the cream scones, the fairy cakes. Everything. They have all been lovely. Have I told you yet Edna, how grateful the whole group is to you? Some of us are even thinking that we might start going to church . Why? Because you are so kind. You have reminded us what being a Christian is all about. It is as if by loving your cakes, we are being drawn to a higher and deeper form of love.

Now all this will end. We can expect no more cakes. But the memory of them will ever remain in our hearts.

Yours
Peter

Chapter 4
Locke's Bucket Diet

which explains the connection between what comes in and what goes out.

John Locke

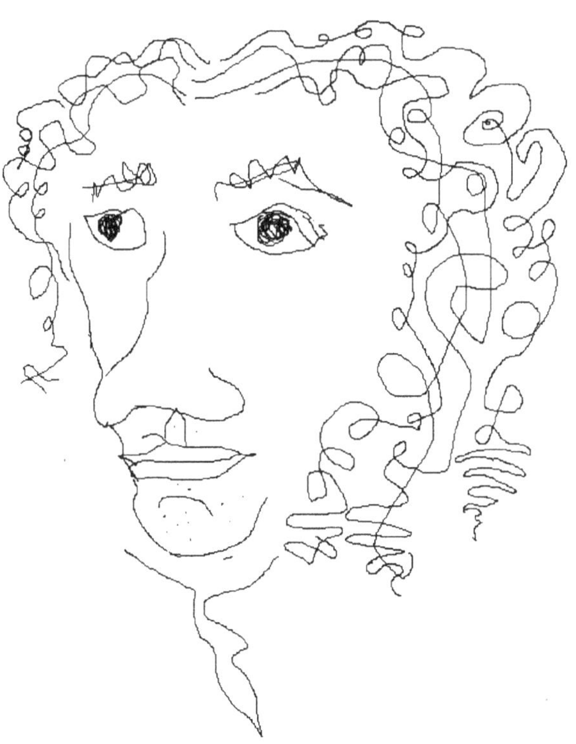

John Locke is the philosophical founder of the greatest nation on earth. I mean of course the USA, which has a constitution inspired by his defence of human rights. Locke, in other words, is a philosopher of democracy. But he also has plenty to say about dieting, more in fact than any other philosopher. Other philosophers may explain or hint at how dieting is part of their bigger picture of the world, but they tend to say little or nothing about the *minutia* of how to diet. Locke, however, tells you exactly what you should and should not eat, and how often you should eat it.

If you have read about The Diet of Pigs in Chapter Two, alarm bells should be ringing at this point. Plato has shown us that democrats tend to eat too much. And as we have seen, the USA is not just the greatest nation on earth, it is also one of the fattest. So you might well wonder whether a democratic philosopher like Locke is going to be very helpful in teaching us how to diet. You are probably thinking: 'Sure Locke may have lots of advice, but is it any good? Might it even be harmful because by helping to make the USA a *democracy*, Locke has ultimate responsibility for making millions of Americans overweight?' These are very fair questions. Indeed, if Locke were alive today a consortium of overweight Americans would probably come together in a class-action suit to sue him.

Locke on Trial

The case for the prosecution is simple: (a) Democracy makes you fat. (b) John Locke more or less invented American democracy. Therefore, (c) John Locke makes you fat. If I were a defense lawyer, how would I respond to this charge? In answer, I think I would simply repeat, in laborious detail, all of Locke's dieting rules. In 1693 Locke wrote a book about how to raise children where he referred again and again to dieting. The book is frankly a bit offensive to any parent. Locke (himself a bachelor) says that most parents literally spoil their children rotten by giving them too much meat and too many sweets and other luscious delicacies and not enough proper food. Having condemned about 90% of parents as pretty useless, Locke becomes even more offensive when you start to realise that he is not really talking about children at all, or rather he thinks that his dieting rules *apply just as well to adults* and that most adults are, in effect, simply a larger version of a spoiled child alternately whinging for food, refusing to eat their vegetables, and gulping down all kinds of rich, fatty, spicy, sweet and salty foods that are bad for them. The only thing that stops most adults from eating too much, says Locke, is that they are too poor to afford it; as soon as they have enough money to gorge themselves with food, they do.

Locke's solution to all this is to do as the ancient Romans did. Eat nothing all day, he says, or if you must, just carry around a lump of bread and a few raisons and munch on them. Then have a meal in the evening; one meal a day is generally enough. Sometimes Locke lets up a bit and allows that you can have two or three meals, but he insists that they be very plain. Meat should be served up 'without other sauce than hunger.' No salt or sugar should be added. Chew your food thoroughly.

Locke also gives an intriguing suggestion for the mind body diet. He says that we should try and *fool* our bodies by having not regular meals, but rather *irregular* meals. Our stomach, he says, comes to expect a regular meal and starts complaining when it is due. If we do not have a regular meal, then it will not know when to complain.

From these observations, Locke gives a summing up of his dieting recommendations.

(1) Eat dry bread for breakfast.

(2) Eat plain unadorned food, for 'dinner' and 'supper.'

(3) The times of these two meals are to be varied constantly across the afternoon and evening so as to keep your stomach guessing.

(4) The kind of food you can eat includes (a) lots of vegetables, (b) a small amount of plain cooked meat or fish, and (c) 'flummery' ,'milk pottage' and 'water-gruel,' or in today's terms: stew, soup and porridge.

(5) If you get hungry in between, you can eat as much dry bread as you like (brown bread is better). The bread should be dry because though nourishing it does not taste very nice.

(6) Locke adds that a child following this diet (he is still ostensibly talking about children) should be allowed to wash the bread down with as much beer as he or she can stomach.*

Pointing all this out would surely be enough to acquit Locke of the charge that he made millions of American's fat.

'Ladies and gentlemen of the jury,' I would conclude, 'how could someone who repeatedly extols the virtues of eating nothing but dry bread all day *possibly* be accused of making people overweight? Anyone who follows John Locke's advice will end up with the lean physique of a tough Roman soldier. This prosecution is outrageous. Not only is my client innocent, but he is doing everything in his power to help his readers lose weight and look great. To accuse John Locke, of all people, of making people fat is probably the most unjust charge ever to be brought before a court!'

---

* To avoid any misunderstanding, and efforts to sue me on the part of angry parents claiming '*he said in his book that I should feed my child unlimited quantities of beer,*' it is worth reiterating that Locke's advice is really for adults.

I think I would get Locke off the hook with a speech like that. However, verdicts in an adversarial legal system are not really based on who tells the truth but rather on who can lie the most persuasively. My client might be innocent in the eyes of the law, but my heart I would, nonetheless, feel that John Locke was guilty.

To try and explain this let me start with an analogy. The father of communism is Karl Marx, and if he were placed before a court, he would have far more to answer for than people getting fat. Under communism countless millions of innocent people have been sent to forced labour camps, tortured and killed. To defend Marx, it would be easy to say, 'Oh no! That was not Karl Marx's fault at all. *His* vision of communism was full of people being all happy and peaceful and creative, not like those horrid countries with their nasty dictators.' Now this defence is superficially true, but at a deeper level it is false. If you advocate a system that repeatedly ends in appalling atrocities, it is no good saying plaintively 'but I told everyone to be *nice* to each other.' There is obviously something about the system—your system—that *causes* all these terrible things to happen, and they happen regardless of you saying that in your fond imagination everything will be wonderful.

Now let us go back to John Locke's advocacy of democracy. In a democracy everyone has the freedom to eat too much, and most of them do. And just as Locke predicted, as a democracy becomes richer so more and more of its citizens gain weight, exactly as has happened in America. It is no good Locke saying: 'It's nothing to do with me. I *told* them to eat wholesome meals and limit snacks to dry bread,' because you know and I know and *he* knows that there is *no way* that people are going to take *any notice* of a diet like that.

They are not going to do it now in the twenty first century and I very much doubt that they were going to do it back in 1693 either.

Incidentally, I think this is why Locke aimed his diet at children. He knew perfectly well that adults would find living off plain food and dry bread so unappealing that they would refuse to follow such a diet, but he hoped that they would force their children to follow it. In a way there is some sense in Locke's general advice that children should eat healthy food and avoid snacks. You can smoke, and still hope that if—between puffs—you firmly tell your children that smoking is bad, that they will do as you say and not as you do. Similarly, you can be overweight and still try to help your children acquire healthy eating habits that they will hopefully carry into adulthood. However, as Locke himself pointed out, this is hardly ideal because if your children see you tucking in to sweets and biscuits every day they will start to wonder why all they get is dried bread.

By the time I had reached this point in my research, I was ready to abandon Locke. He could say all he liked about munching on bread and raisons, but it still was his democracy that had made us all fat in the first place. Then I came across a little passage that made me start in amazement, utter amazement. It was so simple, so brilliant, so obvious. It was the answer to everything.

Locke's Amazing Idea

'OK,' said Angie. 'Let's see if I've got this thing right.'

Angie was the smartest of the Guinea Pigs, so I had decided to explain Locke to her first. If I could get Angie on my side, then all the others would follow. I listened as she counted off the points I had made on her fingers.

'Point One. John Locke has given us democracy, which makes us fat.'

'Right.'

'Point Two. He has given us a diet which, while theoretically feasible, is for all practical purposes completely useless for adults because they will refuse to follow it.'

'Correct.'

Point Three. The diet is of dubious value for children, because if we won't follow it, how can we expect them to?'

'Exactly.'

'OK. So Point Four, why have you just wasted my time telling me all this if it is basically useless? Why consider John Locke at all if his diet is no good?'

When Angie asked this I could barely stop myself from smiling; I tingled with excitement.

'Angie,' I said, 'I have something to confess. I have been keeping a secret from you.'

'What?'

I wriggled my thumb teasingly at Angie,

'You're forgetting Point Five. John Locke said *something else* about dieting, something that I've not yet told you. He had an amazing idea! It is something that is incredibly easy to do, and it is something that is fantastically effective at making you lose weight. It costs almost nothing. It requires very little effort. Follow this one simple technique and I think—I am tempted to say I *guarantee*—that you will lose weight and look great at an incredible rate!'

'Well, what is it then?'

'Locke's idea is brilliant, it is extraordinary and I am *bursting* to tell you about it. But I'm not going to tell you. Not yet. I want to whet your appetite a bit more first by telling you one of the fabulous things about Locke's diet. *You can eat whatever you like and still lose weight!*'

Angie snorted contemptuously.

'How many times have I read that claim in diet books and magazines? And it's not true. I know it's not true because I've tried the diets. I'm disappointed in you Peter. Saying you can eat as much as you like and lose weight is a lie, a flagrant, preposterous lie.'

'Angie,' I said solemnly, 'I swear that with John Locke's wonderful dieting idea, it really is true, literally true. You can eat as much as you like and still lose weight. Because this one idea of Locke's provides the most astonishingly effective diet you can imagine.'

'This sounds worse and worse,' said Angie incredulously. 'It's like one of those books that promises to tell you the secret of how to get rich and then, after stringing you along, ends with three ordinary greedy little words: "become a landlord." Whatever this dieting idea is, I bet it will be dumb. Now hurry up and tell me it.'

'Oh, all right.'

'Well then?'

'Can't I say about how exciting it is a bit more?'

'No.'

'Can I make a sort of drum roll noise to announce it?'

'No. Just tell me what it is.'

I took a deep breath and then, in a quiet but intense voice, told Angie the secret.

'Poo once a day.'

'Poo?'

'Yes.'

'Once a day?'

'Yes. Locke said: "*Once in four and twenty hours, I think is enough; and no body, I guess, will think it too much.*" '

'So *that* is John Locke's "wonderful" idea?'

'Yes!'

'Oh.'

John Harington and the Democratic Metabolism

I had let the cat out of the bag and it was obvious that Angie was disappointed by it. It is possible that you, the reader, may also be feeling a little let down, and perhaps some explanation is called for. OK. To understand the brilliance of Locke's idea, it helps to realise how going to the lavatory once a day is closely connected to his democratic political philosophy. To do that we first need to remember Descartes's distinction between the mind and body. According to Descartes, the problem with dieting is how to get the mind to control the body. Locke argues the opposite; the real problem is how to get the body to control the mind, or head. Now to explain this, we can bring in someone else, a man called John Harington, who lived about a hundred years before Locke.

Harington is famous for a little rhyme that sums up a big political-philosophical problem. The rhyme goes like this:

Treason doth never prosper, what's the reason?
For if it prosper, none dare call it treason.

In a way this is a joke: if someone manages to becomes king by killing the old king, then no one has the courage to complain. Instead everyone goes round saying 'things are fine,' and that it was quite right and proper that the old king was smothered with a pillow or impaled with a red hot poker or whatever. But there is more to the rhyme than that, because it implies that whatever the king says is law (none dare call it treason). The king, the head of state, is at the top and everyone else—and this it is significant—is at the *bottom*. So all the laws come down from the king at the top to the bottom, and that the only way for those at the bottom to change the law is by a violent attack on the king.

Locke thought this was a rotten political system and wanted to change it around. Instead of absolute monarchy—we might as well call it tyranny—in which the people were bossed around by the king the whole time and could only change things by violence, Locke's democratic alternative was that the people at the bottom would somehow control the king (or government) at the top. If the people at the bottom wanted the laws to change, then the king/government at the top would get the message and would peacefully change the law.

If we now go back to dieting, the king is like our head and the people are like our body. If we are going to have a democratic metabolism, the body is not going to spend its time being bossed around by the head. Instead, the body is going to tell the head what to do. But how? How can it get its message to the head? Sometimes the body sends a message by violent 'treason.' If you suffer a heart attack, that is a pretty strong and violent message from the body to the head that you had better shape up and follow a low fat diet. But there is no need for the message to be violent. The simple peaceful way of sending a message from the body to the head, from bottom to top, is by (a) pooing, or by (b) not pooing. What's the message?

> (a) Every time you poo, your bottom is telling your head: 'I want more food. I have more space. Fill me up!'

(b) Every time you *don't* poo, it is saying: 'I'm full, don't stuff any more food in.'

So if you poo less, then you will eat less too.

Another way of explaining the genius of Locke's idea is that it reverses our usual view of cause and effect. Instead of thinking:

The more you eat, the more you poo.

you realise:

The more you poo, the more you eat.

In other words, it is not eating that determines how much we poo, it is pooing that determines how much we eat. And that means that if we can just get our pooing right, then everything else in our diet will *automatically* come right too. Providing only that we poo correctly, we will not even need to *think* about what we eat. Losing weight will follow as day follows night. We will lose weight without even realising we are on a diet.

It is often the mark of a great idea that as soon as you say it, it sounds obvious. And what could be more obvious than this? Locke's poo-control diet explains, at a stroke, the mystery of the millions of people who, without being particularly athletic, still manage to have wonderfully slim bodies (even though they are often surrounded by other people who are overweight). If you ask someone who appears to be 'naturally' slim like this what their 'secret' is, they never really know what to say. The fact is that most of them are not spending their time counting the calories or doing any special diet, they have simply learned poo control. And because this control has become a habit, they probably do not even realise what they are doing. Even if they *do* realise, they are not going to tell you. Imagine, for example, sitting in an open plan office and saying to a colleague:

'I envy you being so slim. How *do* you manage it?'

They are hardly likely to reply:

'I have learned to control my poo.'

As this would be embarrassing, not least because it would imply:

'And you haven't.'

So instead they will make something up about how they are dieting, or deflect the question with a complement about you in return, and you will be none the wiser.

Before we leave John Harington, you should know that there is one more thing that he is famous for. Harington invented the water closet. The toilet or 'WC' that we sit on today is essentially the same as that designed by Harington back in 1596. It is testimony to the genius of John Locke that he grasped, or at least intuited, the disastrous impact that this invention would have upon his democratic project.

The Bucket

I want to get back to Angie for a minute, because—and this is typical of Angie—she did not just laugh at Locke's poo diet or dismiss it because it sounded odd. Instead she asked a question that went right to the heart of whether or not it would work:

'What if I want to poo *more* than once a day. What then?'

Now Locke gave detailed instructions on how to overcome this problem.* He admitted, it would take several months constant practice to get it right, so we will not go into that. Instead, I am able to make my own modest contribution to following Locke's diet, by sharing with you a much simpler, quicker way of reaching the desired end. It is a technique that works within a day or two, and I know it works, because I have tried it myself.

I have tried to avoid discussing my own diets because his book is not, in any way shape or form, about me; it is entirely about the great philosophers and my job as the author is simply to draw out their insights before slipping unobtrusively into the background. However, I want to make an exception here and mention my own experience because it is so useful for keeping to Locke's diet.

When I was younger I used to go primitive camping in Wales for two weeks every summer with my parents, brother and three sisters. For those two weeks I would eat like a horse; we all did. But at the end of the two weeks, it did not matter how much I had eaten. I had invariably lost weight; we had all lost weight. Why? The answer *seemed* obvious: it was because of all the walking, swimming, surfing, and outdoor games we were playing. And for many years that is what I believed.

But things are not always what they seem.

These camping trips are now a thing of the past. My parents, my brother, and one of my sisters have all brought houses in the area where we once pitched up our tents. My sister's house is a dream house. It has three fully equipped

---

* If you would like to follow up Locke's advice on this matter, read his account of 'Costiveness' in *Some Thoughts Concerning Education.*

bathrooms, which I think helps tell you what kind of house it is, and a couple of years ago, I went to stay there. I walked, I swam, I swimhiked, I surfed and I played outdoor games all day. I also ate like a horse, but this was OK, I thought, because of all the exercise I was doing.

At the end of the holiday, I was shocked to discover that I had gained weight. What had gone wrong? Why had I gained weight when I stayed in a house when I had always lost weight when I stayed in a tent? Strange as the answer may seem, the problem was my sister's lavatories. There were just too many of them and they were too comfortable. It meant I spent the whole time pooing, and of course, the more I pooed, the more I ate. Why, therefore, did I lose weight when we went primitive camping? Until I read Locke, the answer to this question simply became a mystery. After I had read him the scales fell from my eyes. It *wasn't* all the swimming, the surfing the walks and the games after all. It was 'the bucket.'

'The bucket' was our camping toilet. A short distance away from the main tent my father would dig a trench about eighteen inches wide, three foot long and three foot deep. He would pile up the earth by the side of the trench and stick the spade in the top of the pile. Next to the trench he would pitch the toilet tent. Inside the tent was a bucket, a roll of toilet paper, a bottle of disinfectant, a torch, and some resident bluebottles. When you needed to poo, you would (1) sit on the bucket, (2) empty the poo from the bucket into the trench, (3) clean the bucket with toilet paper and put that in the trench too, (4) cover it all up with a thin layer of earth, and (5) head back to the main tents to wash your hands from one of the water containers. My mother would also (6) sterilise the bucket with the disinfectant, but I am not sure how often the rest of us would bother.

Once you got used to it, visiting the bucket was fine. But it was never exactly enjoyable, and none of us went there more than we had to. I would quickly adjust to pooing about once every 36 hours. And as Locke explains, this meant that although I was eating until I was full, I was actually eating less than I normally did.

The conclusion is obvious: if you want to lose weight, poo in a bucket.

We can now go back to Angie's question, 'what if I want to poo *more* than once a day?' Providing you use a bucket, the answer is simple: 'you *won't* want to.' The great thing about the bucket diet is that *this question does not even arise*.

Following Locke's Diet

There are two basic methods to choose from for Locke's diet. Either will work although the first is the most effective, which is why I recommend it

Option 1 (recommended)

To follow Locke's diet, you simply need to recreate, insofar as is possible, the conditions of 'the bucket' in you own home. With sufficient garden, it may well be possible that you can recreate them exactly. This is the ideal, and if you are serious about losing weight and looking great it is undoubtedly the best diet to follow. Toilet tents can be purchased from any large camping store.

Option 2 (The fall back option)

If you do not own a garden or prefer a gentler dieting method, a fall back option is simply to place a bucket (and appropriate cleaning equipment) next to your lavatory. Whenever you need to do a poo, do not use your WC, use the bucket instead then empty it into your toilet bowl. (Note that there is no need for any guests to know the bucket's purpose, to them, it will simply be the place you happen to keep it.) This, of course, this will not work as well, as it is considerably more comfortable than camping. There is no tent, no bluebottles. You do not need to venture outside. If it is dark you have an electric light. There is no hole to fill with a thin layer of earth, and there is a sink of hot and cold water to hand. But even with all these advantages, you will find that sitting on a bucket is not nearly as comfortable and convenient as a WC, and you will adjust accordingly.

I know you will want to find out how the Guinea Pigs fared on this diet, but first let's go over why the bucket diet is so effective. Back in the sixteenth century everyone's daily experience of going to the toilet was roughly that of primitive camping. However, once Harington had invented the water closet, the incentive to exercise strict control over how frequently we pooed was removed at exactly the time that we most needed its discipline to counter to the spread of democracy with its 'do whatever you feel like' ethos. The rest, as they say, is history. There are details to fill in, of course, but I will leave it to the historians and the statisticians to chart the relationship between the spread of comfortable toilets (outdoors to indoors, hard paper to soft paper and so on) with the demographics of weight gain. Suffice it to say that the spread of democracy plus increasingly comfortable toilets is the lethal cocktail that has lead to the crisis of being overweight. We *like* going to comfortable toilets, and, weak willed democrats that we are, we go again and again. It is ironic that with millions being spent on dieting aids of all kinds it is the humble bucket that can solve the 'obesity crisis' at a stroke. So while John Locke was partly responsible for getting us into this mess he also identified the solution. Indeed, it is my hope that given the huge respect with which Locke is held in the United States that this nation in particular will benefit from the bucket diet.

Incident with Stuart

I was sat in the church hall with Angie, Derek, Jasmine, Stuart and Wendy—who was now elfin slim but who had come to support her husband. I had explained the diet, and we had finished our usual excellent tea, the Vicar's wife (though not the Vicar) having forgiven us. Now came the moment of truth. I went in to the kitchen area and came back with five all-purpose orange plastic buckets. Wendy, of course, did not need one, but the other Guinea Pigs were looking at them with some trepidation, so before handing them out I gave a little speech.

'These buckets are brand new,' I said. 'They are fresh from the hardware store and they are my gift to you. I'm giving them to you because you're not just my Guinea Pigs, you've become my friends, and because I trust you to use them. Also, I think these buckets represent your best shot at losing weight and looking great. Look, we've all been brought up as democrats and philosophically we are all at least partly "liberal." Liberalism is a nice philosophy, much nicer than some of the other stuff. Now Locke isn't the only liberal philosopher, but he's certainly one of the best. So if we can't use Locke to get us to lose weight, then what does that mean? It means that we have to get into other, darker philosophies, the philosophies of the Four Germans. And if you think Locke's diet is strange, wait until you see what *they* suggest!'

The GPs did not look wholly convinced, but I pressed on.

'OK, ladies first. Jasmine!'

I passed Jasmine a bucket. She took it as though I had handed her a slug. I had guessed Jasmine would be reluctant, that was one reason why it had been so important to get Angie on my side beforehand, because I knew Jasmine looked up to her.

'Angie!'

I tried to pass Angie a bucket.

'No,' said Angie.

There was a stunned silence. *I* was stunned. After all the time I had spent explaining Locke's diet to Angie, for her to refuse like that was a bolt from the blue.

'Angie,' I said as gently as I could, 'Do you mind explaining why not?'

'No' said Angie. 'Oh all right, yes, what does it matter? I already poo less than once a day. And hey: I'm fat. I'm sorry Peter, but I just think this whole diet is a load of crap.'

'Well, of course it won't work for everyone, I began, 'I mean, that's the whole point of going through all the different philosophers…'

But Angie wasn't listening, she was just shaking her head and, to my surprise, it was Derek who stepped in to save the session.

'I'll take one,' said Derek, 'No sweat. Fact is, I'm used to it from prison.'

'I didn't know you'd been in prison Derek,' I said politely, though in fact I did.

'Yeah, Cuba,' said Derek. 'Political prisoner.'

From what I understood of the nature of Derek's offence it hardly qualified him as a 'political prisoner.' Derek, however, managed to say it in such a way that suggested that if he was concealing anything, it was that he had been on some kind of James Bond mission. Under the circumstances I let this pass. Thirty seconds earlier Angie had almost scuppered the diet before we had even tried it. Now Derek, had completely changed things around and the bucket had acquired an aura of masculine bravado. Jasmine was looking at him with a smouldering interest, while Stuart quickly said he'd have a bucket too. Angie rolled her eyes but kept her peace.

As if to emphasise his own toughness, Stuart announced that, as things happened, he was going to go and use the bucket right away, and went to the toilet that adjoined the hall, swinging the bucket nonchalantly as he went. Wendy, I think, was quietly proud of him.

It was about five minutes later that we heard the cries of distress. It is tiresome, but in the light of later comments that I was 'too tight fisted to buy extra strength buckets' I want to make it absolutely plain that the bucket did *not* break under Stuart's weight and that he had simply slipped off it somehow and allowed it to overturn. Be that as it may, once Wendy had gone in and extricated him from this situation, he had changed his mind about using it.

This was where it was useful that Wendy was coming to support her husband to lose weight, because with her encouragement we quickly worked out an alternative plan. There was a public lavatory very close to their village home. When Stuart needed to go, he would use that.

A week later Stuart was arrested for loitering. Of course, one can see why if someone is frequently going out of their own home to visit a public lavatory that this might arouse suspicion amongst neighbours and CCTV operators. As for the rest, Angie continued dismissive, and Derek and Jasmine used the buckets only to mix paint and wallpaper glue at Jasmine's flat. However, I retain a strong faith in Locke's method of dieting. So much so that before we conclude Section One of this book, I want to recommend that anyone thoughtful enough to present this book as a gift to someone who might benefit from it, should also provide them with a bucket.

The Bucket Diet in a Nutshell

1. Buy a bucket
2. Poo in it.

Sources

John Locke, *Two Treatises of Government*
John Locke, *Some Thoughts Concerning Education*

Dear Edna,
What can I say? Those were the best home-made biscuits that any of us had _ever_ tasted. And even more importantly, you have forgiven us. The little knock on the door, the tray piled high, the gorgeous wafting aroma. I felt as if … well, I do not think I can adequately explain quite how it makes me feel.
Thank you Edna.

Thank you
Thank you
Peter

Part II
The Four Germans

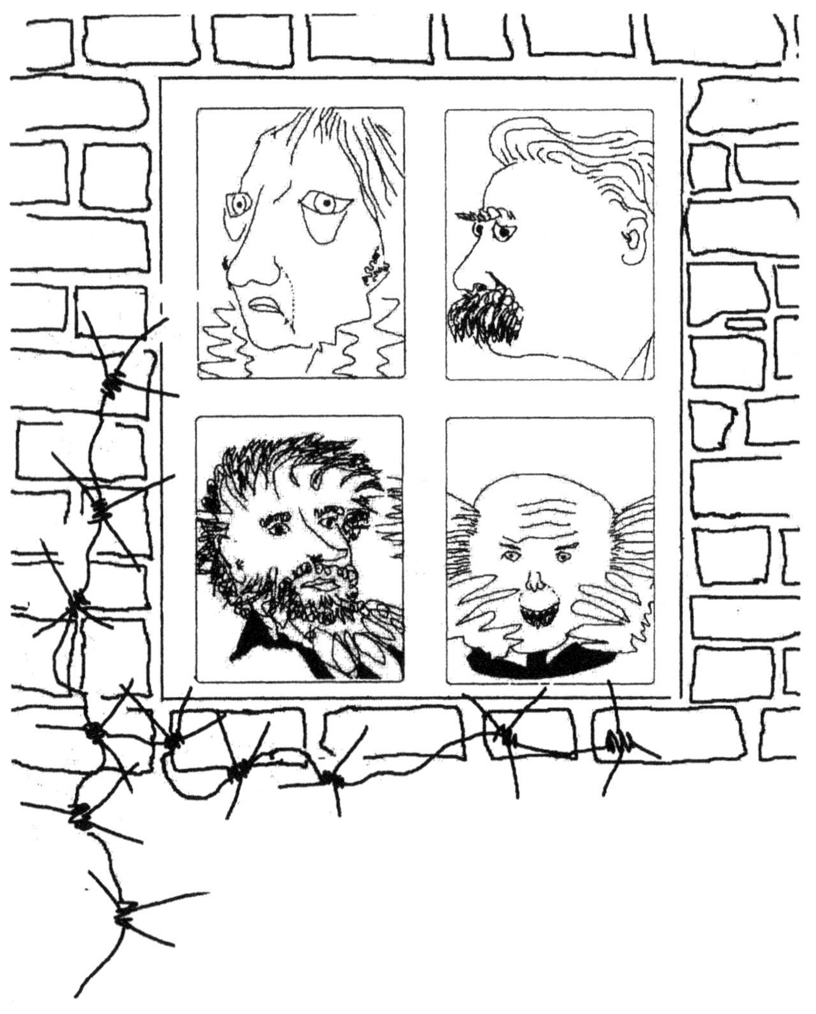

The first thing you notice about the Four Germans is how hairy most of them look. There is Nietzsche with his gigantic moustache staring fixedly at nothing. There is Schopenhauer, bald on top but with his white hair sticking out proudly on each side like an enormous pair of perky ears. And there is Marx with his exorbitant beard, looking half like God, half Father Christmas. Only Hegel, who simply looks despondent, could in any sense be said to appear 'normal.' He is clean shaven and the hair on his head is reasonably neat.

But is this a fair way of proceeding? Surely we are deceived by appearances? Of course people looked rather different over a hundred years ago, but we are interested in their minds, not how they look; underneath all that hair they were no doubt perfectly sensible.

If only that were true! In fact, if only it were true that their looks were *not* deceptive and that the great German philosophers were simply wild and eccentric as well as hairy. The actual truth is infinitely more terrible.

Of course, we all know in a general way what happened. First Schopenhauer introduced a corrosive cynicism into philosophy by announcing that there is no God and that we are all repulsive grubby little creatures and nothing we do matters in the least. (I am not exaggerating, in fact I am toning him down a bit.) Then Marx turned half the world into communists, Nietzsche invented the Nazis, and before we know it we have World War II, the Holocaust and the Gulag.

What of Hegel, the normal looking one? What was his role in all this? It is hard to tell. Hegel was writing at the beginning of the nineteenth century, a bit earlier than the rest of them. He had an acknowledged influence on Marx, who began his philosophical career as a 'young Hegelian' and it is pretty obvious that he influenced the others too, even though Schopenhauer said he hated him and Nietzsche pretended to ignore him. Some think that Hegel was misunderstood by the later philosophers who, for all their imposingly hairy features, were actually rather weak minded and never really worked out what he meant. Read Hegel aright, they say, and you will not *necessarily* end up wanting to kill millions of innocent people. I tend to think this myself, which is why one or two of Hegel's ideas have already been allowed to creep in to some of our diets. Others say that despite his relatively normal appearance, Hegel is the nastiest philosopher of the lot.

In any event, you can see why, all in all, I felt a bit cautious about introducing the Four Germans to the Guinea Pigs. If they had been able to lose weight with help from Bergson, Plato, Hobbes, Descartes and Locke, then we would have stayed safe amongst philosophers who were essentially reasonable people. Once we strayed in amongst the Four Germans, goodness knows what would happen.

Reader be warned; you too are about to enter dangerous ground. Imagine this book is a wildlife park where, guided by me, you can wander freely amongst the animals. So far we have been spending our time in the 'family enclosure' with Hobbes the tortoise, Locke the lemur and Bergson the bunny. Now we are at the double gate to another enclosure. At the entrance it says:

Beware
Dangerous Animals

'Yes, and they're not joking, best stay outside...' I begin, but it is already too late, your interest is peaked and you push on through the gates to see what you can find within. Immediately an ugly looking piebald creature stands up on its long legs, sniffs, and starts loping up towards you. It is Schopenhauer the wild hunting dog.

'Oh, how cute! Look at those sticking out ears!'

'He's not cute!' I yell. 'Keep away from him!'

But it is no use; the exit is already cut off by Marx the grizzly bear. All I can do is grab a large stick and hastily follow. Oh reader please be warned! The Four Germans are not safe, tame philosophers. If you go any further into Section Two, goodness knows what will happen to you. True, you may come out of the experience having lost weight and looking great, but at what cost? Your looks have changed for the better on the outside, but what of the changes *within*? What mad visions running through your mind? What awful thoughts unleashed? Beware reader, I say again: Beware.

Beware
Dangerous Philosophers

Chapter 5
Marx's Revolutionary Diet

which explains why having less weight makes you more human.

Karl Marx playing hangman

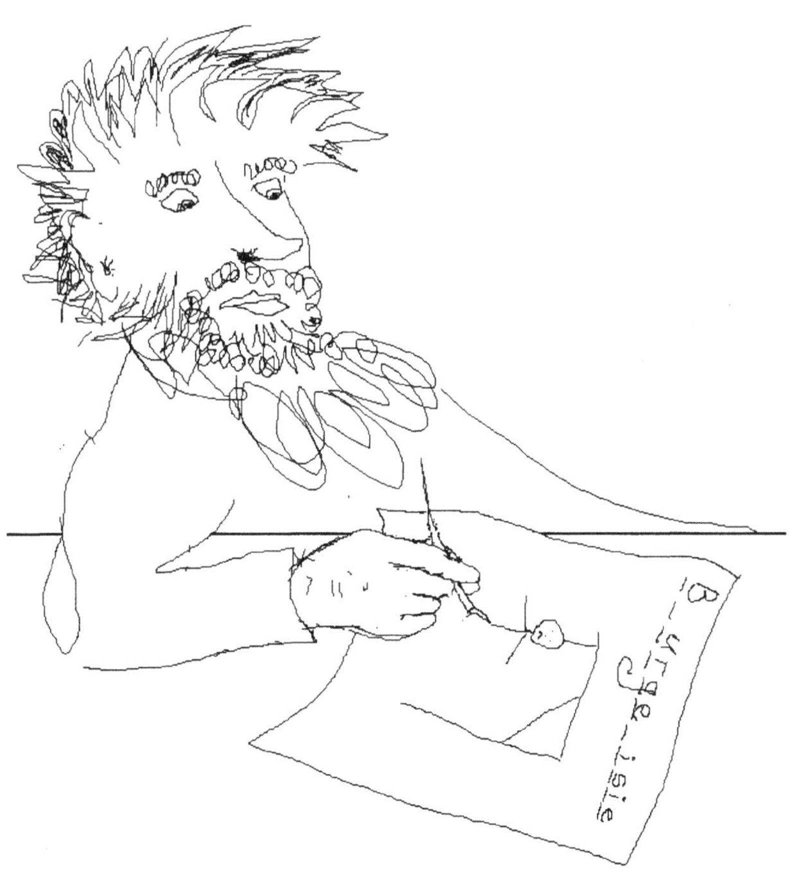

Karl Marx says that society is basically made up two big classes. One is the *bourgeois* or capitalist class, meaning the bosses. The other is the *proletariat* or working class, meaning all the people who are bossed around. These classes do not get along, and in fact are always fighting against each other. At the moment the capitalists, who have almost all the wealth, are winning. The only way in which the working class can really improve their downtrodden lives is by having a revolution, taking *all* the wealth off the capitalists and sharing it out. And if the capitalists don't like it, Marx says, then hang them from the lampposts and see how they like *that*.

At this point you may be thinking:

'Yes. This is all very philosophical, but what has it got to do with me dieting?'

The answer depends on how you make a living. If you are one of the bosses then the question is in sense academic, because Karl Marx does not want you to lose weight, he wants to you to be hanged. If, however, you make your living by earning wages, then it has *everything* to do with you. Wage earners like you are proletarians, and are overweight because they—you—are *miserable*. When the working class have a revolution they will stop being miserable and hence stop being overweight.

There are many more workers than there are capitalists, so why hasn't there been a revolution already? Well, according to Marxist revolutionaries there is a capitalist plot going on and it is this.

(1) Give the workers a *little bit* more money

(2) Give them a *little bit* more free time to spend their money

(3) Tell them *lots* of lies.

'That,' the cunning capitalists think, 'ought to be enough to prevent a revolution and save our necks' And indeed, until now it has been enough. With a bit more money and time and lots of lies the workers have *not* staged a revolution. What have they done instead? You've guessed it; they have grown fat.

The working class has been given enough money to eat too much and enough time to eat it. This is partly because the capitalists have realised that *someone* has to go to the shops they own, buy the stuff they make and *consume* it, else they will all go bankrupt. But it is their lies that have really saved the day for the capitalists. One lie is that you 'need' employers to give you a job (actually they need you). A second lie is that chief executives and bankers get paid millions of pounds every year because they are tremendously talented (actually they are not talented, just powerful). A third lie is the Christian idea that justice will be served in heaven, so you just have to put up with being pushed around on the earth. That is why Marx said 'Religion is the opium of the people': it acts like a debilitating drug that deprives believers of any get-up-and-go. These lies have been tremendously successful at turning the revolutionary energy of the working class in on itself. Instead of attacking the capitalists, the proletariat have attacked their own bodies by becoming overweight.

You may now be thinking a 'Frequently Asked Question.'

FAQ *I am working class and fat. Does this mean that I have to wait for a revolution to lose weight?*

No! You do *not* need to wait for a revolution. By following the revolutionary diet you can lose weight and look great *even under the rotten capitalist system.* The great thing about this diet is that once you have seen through all lies and realise what is really going on, there is no need to wait for a revolution to lose weight. It is the *anticipation* of the revolution, the build-up, that will have an incredible impact on your diet. While you prepare to transform society, you will find that you are transforming your body. Striving to free your class from their oppressors will quickly lead you to shed your surplus flesh and reform your physique in a heroic mould. All the energy that had turned inwards into endless consumption and self-destructive fattening will flow outwards in a healthy hatred of the class enemy! Have you seen photos of the incredibly athletic, healthy, vigorous and generally great looking workers in the old USSR? Well that is what people looked like back then under communism. And that is what *you* will look like.

There are at least three ways of taking the revolutionary diet forward. The first is not, I think, the most likely Marxist method to lose weight; its appeal is likely to be quite narrow as it requires quite a lot of commitment. However, it will undoubtedly work for the right kind of person, and as that person may be you it is worth explaining. It is called the cell diet.

Class Conflict under Capitalism

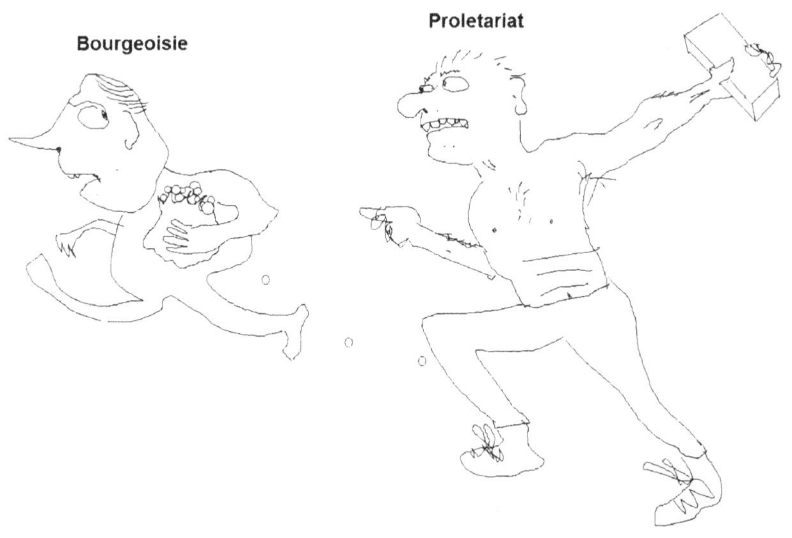

The Cell Diet

The cell diet is nothing to do with cellulose or cellulite. Rather, it requires that you actively prepare for a communist revolution. To do this you need to locate and join a communist (or 'anti-capitalist') cell. (There is almost sure to be one in your area, just ask at your local library or check the internet.) Exactly what you do in the cell will vary. You may find yourself jetting all over the world to attend environmental protests. You may find yourself performing plays—apparently innocent but which carry a hidden communist message—for classes of school children. But whatever you are doing, you will find that you are losing weight! Your energy is being redirected. No longer are you a consumer but a revolutionary with a real purpose in life. Your whole attitude to life changes, and your body changes too. (Also, being part of a cell is a great way to make new friends with fellow activists and undercover police officers.) So this is potentially a highly effective diet, but if you do not particularly like the hours of work involved and the risk of being locked up, there is another revolutionary diet to try: the shed diet.

The Shed Diet

I call this 'the shed diet' not because you will shed fat, although you will, but because you can do it in a shed. In this respect the shed diet is much easier than the cell diet. There is no need to associate with wild eyed anarchists with rings through their noses and sordid agent provocateurs; you just have to take yourself off down the garden to your little wooden hut. In fact, just about anyone can do it, particularly as you do not even need a shed to do it in.

'What,' Marx asks, 'makes us human?' His answer is that *we make things when we do not need to.* Birds build nests so they can lay their eggs in them and bees build their hives to store honey, but no animal ever makes anything just for fun. Only we do. Imagine a small boy and girl on a beach happily absorbed in building a sandcastle or a dam. These children, says Marx, are not being childish; they are becoming human.

Under capitalism we are constantly making things that we do not need: we are overloaded with cars, gizmos, knick knacks, TV shows, bureaucratic forms, incessant pop music and—of course—vast amounts of food, far more than we can possibly eat without becoming overweight. The problem with this is not that we *have* all this unnecessary stuff. No, the true problem is that the capitalist system takes all the fun out of *making* it. It completely ruins the pleasure to be got from creating unnecessary things, and in fact turns it into a pain. Marx explains how the pleasure of making things becomes horrible with a sort of paradox. Although the great majority of work under capitalism is wholly unnecessary, we *need* to do it. This is not because it actually needs doing but simply because we need a job if we are to earn any money. The capitalist takes advantage this fact to make sure that we are miserable while we work by bossing us around to make us work harder, and insisting that we make everything in exactly the same way until it gets mind numbingly boring.

Now we come to another paradox (Marx liked paradoxes). As we have seen, animals only do things when they need to do them. This means that because we humans *need* to go to work to help to create unnecessary things, we feel no better than an animal in our jobs. Work, which ought to be making us feel more human, is actually making us feel less than human.

How do can we get to feel human again? We only feel human when we are back at home, away from work. But the activities we do at home are things that we genuinely *need* to do. They are also things that we share doing with animals, like reproducing, excreting and consuming, or in other words having sex, going to the toilet and eating. To make these animal-activities seem more human, we start doing them *when we don't need to.* We have sex when we don't need to. As we know from John Locke, we go to the toilet when we don't need to. *And we eat when we don't need to.*

OK. If that just about sums up your life, *don't worry.* There are *millions* of people who are in *exactly* the same position as you. And the good news is that there is a simple solution at hand: get a shed, and start making things inside it. What to make? Well, you could paint pictures, engineer miniature working traction engines, carve antler-headed walking sticks. The possibilities, in fact, are almost endless, but the principles are these:

(1) Keep it separate from your job

(2) Do it for fun.

(3) Do not be too repetitive: make things differently, make each one unique.

Once you start enjoy making things you will discover that you lose weight. If you need convincing of this, examine people who expend time and energy in their sheds working at a really creative hobby. Very few of them, you will notice, are overweight, and even those that are don't seem to care very much. They love what they do. They feel that they are using all their abilities; feel that they have made a great choice of hobby; when they hit a problem they are excited and interested about how to solve it. They feel really satisfied and absorbed when they are making something and proud when they have finished it. If you could hear inside their hearts what they were feeling as they worked, it would be a joyful happy song, perhaps the Hi-Ho! Hi-Ho! song of the seven dwarfs.

Variants on the shed diet turn up in the überdiet and the love diet and I thoroughly recommend it: it works and it has *no unpleasant side-effects*. However, the truly revolutionary diet I have saved until last. It is called the strike diet, and provided only that you follow its one simple rule, I *promise* that you will lose weight.

The Strike Diet

I am not going to tell you the one simple rule of the strike diet just yet, because first I want you to understand its deeper philosophical context. To do this we need to know a couple more things about Marx's call for revolution. (1) He was totally contemptuous of anyone who thought that the workers could get out of the mess they were in little by little, bit by bit with things gradually getting better. That, Marx said was a hopeless way to go about things. A revolution to uproot everything was only way to succeed. (2) As well as the two classes of bourgeoisie and proletariat, there is a third class who are always getting in the way of a revolution and ruining it. This class is called the lumpenproletariat.

It is rather difficult to pin down exactly who Marx means by the lumpenproletariat. They are obviously bad, because they are on the wrong side. Marx describes them as 'the bribed tool of reactionary intrigue', and as 'scum'. But exactly how the lumpenproletariat are different from the ordinary proletariat is a puzzle. Some say that they are the poorest workers, translating the word lumpen as ragged to make 'ragged-proletariat'. This might seem likely because Marx sometimes links the lumpenproletariat to tramps, beggars and the 'surplus population' who cannot find a job. The problem is that the lumpenproletariat also include gamblers, novelists and brothel madams, who are all quite rich. So if they are not the ragged-proletariat, who are they? The answer is simple. The lumpenproletariat are members of the proletariat who are lumpy. In other words, they are fat. More precisely they are covered in a lump of *surplus* fat.

As soon as it is realised that for 'lumpenproletariat' we can read fat-proletariat, then everything starts to fall in to place. Why has there not been a revolution in the USA, the world's most advanced capitalist state, where most people are members of the proletariat? Because, according to official statistics, most of them are also fat. Overweight people have never, in the whole of human history, staged a revolution of any sort. At most they may have joined in afterwards, when the fighting was over. To protect the capitalist system, the bourgeoisie have done a brilliant thing. By making workers fat, they have turned the proletariat into their own class enemy.*

The Transformation of the Working Class

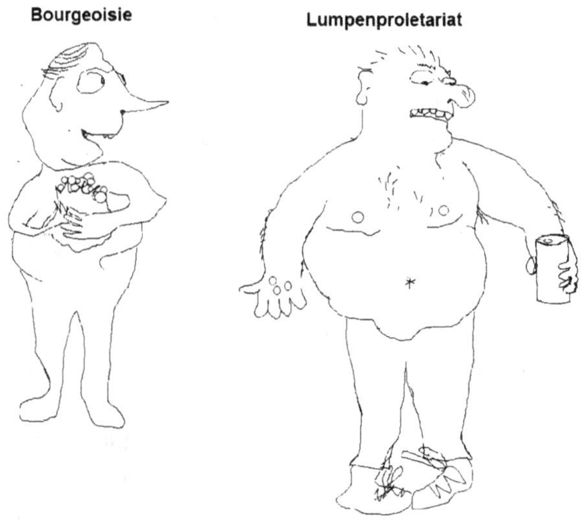

---

* It just so happens that I am an expert on what Marx means by the lumpenproletariat, and it is actually a little more complicated than how I explain it here. If you want to read a more scholarly account of them you can consult my articles '*Utopia* and the Lumpenproletariat' *Review of Politics* 1988, and 'Marx's Analysis of the French Class Structure,' *Theory and Society* 1993, or my book *The People and the Mob* 1992.

It might appear somewhat insulting for overweight working class readers to be told that they are members of the lumpenproletariat. But actually this is both exciting and incredibly important, because it tells you where you are at, and what you want to become. You are *at* the lumpenproletariat, but you want to *become* one of the proletariat who, as I have mentioned, have fantastic bodies. So what do you need to do? The answer is obvious, get rid of your *lump*. How? The answer is implicit in Marx's rejection of reform for revolution. It is no use, says Marx, trying to have slow step-by-step change. You have to go for broke, pull out all the stops and go all the way, at once. If we apply this insight to dieting we end up with the following one simple rule.

Marx's one simple rule for his revolutionary diet is this:

If you want to go an a really effective diet, you must eat *nothing at all.*

It really is as simple as that.

How long should you eat nothing for? *There is no set answer.* You just continue to eat nothing until your surplus fat has gone, and quite how long this will take depends on how lumpen you are.

After a while, there are one or two side effects associated with not eating anything at all, which I will not bore you with except to mention that beyond a certain point they include the risk of death. But most of these side effects are the result of starvation, and as long has you have a good layer of fat around you, you are not going to starve, because your body will eat that. And as soon as your surplus fat has been consumed, you can start eating through your mouth again.

So the strike diet gets its name from going on a food strike, like a hunger strike, and as is often the case in hunger strikes, there is a political reason behind it, because you are waging a kind of battle within your own body between the proletariat and the lumpenproletariat.

You may think: 'I'm not doing that diet. It is far too radical!' But before your reject it, out of hand, think twice. How long have you been trying various little by little step-by-step diets? Weeks? Months? Years? And how many of them have worked? If the answer is 'None of them,' then as far as you are concerned, Marx was right: it is just as hopeless to try and gradually lose weight as it is to get rid of capitalism gradually. And if he was right about *that*, then might he not also be right about the strike diet?

Derek goes on Strike

When I told the Guinea Pigs about the Strike Diet, they were not particularly keen on the idea, and launched into various 'health and safety' objections: What if they ran out of some vital vitamin and caught scurvy? What if they fainted from lack of food while driving an articulated lorry down the motorway? and so on.

The exception was Derek. He was already predisposed to like Marx as someone who attacked 'the system,' and seemed genuinely interested in the revolutionary diet plan offered by his philosophy. In the midst of an emotional speech by Angie about the dangers of anorexia he broke in with a perceptive comment:

'All this stuff about how eating nothing's going to kill you. It's all just bourgeois lies.' Then in a devil-may-care way he announced, 'To me it makes sense, and I'm going to do it.'

In the stunned silence that followed, Derek carefully and deliberately ate a chocolate biscuit. Then he glanced at his watch. 'Starting now.'

'Don't Derek! said Angie urgently, 'Think what you're doing! Stop before it's too late!' She turned to me indignantly, 'How could you Peter? Don't you know the risks…' and started on about the problems faced by teenaged girls with low self-worth who starved themselves.

'I appreciate what you're saying Ange,' said Derek, 'But basically, that's what life's about: taking risks. And, sometimes, you've just got to do something.'

'I'd do the strike diet too' explained Stuart (when Derek was acting tough, Stuart also liked to act tough). 'But I don't think I'd better,' he continued, 'because Wendy wouldn't like it if I died.'

Jasmine was looking more and more upset, and now her eyes started to fill with tears.

'Don't Derek,' she said softly, 'I don't want you to…' Jasmine left the sentence unfinished.

Derek grasped her hand. 'I'll be fine Jasmine,' he said. He gave her a smile, outwardly cheerful, while underneath the surface one sensed an inexpressible sadness. It was a bit like a spitfire pilot saying goodbye to his wife or girlfriend as he was about to take to the air in the Battle of Britain.

I had no concerns at all about Derek. This was partly because, as I have said, anyone with fat to spare does not actually stop eating when they stop eating, they just start eating their fat. And it was partly because, judging by his past form, Derek was certain to cheat in any event.

Meanwhile Angie was busily fiddling with her mobile and started reading from some ridiculous list of what happens when you stop eating that she had found on the internet.

'Nervousness, irritability, fainting fits, kidney failure, hypothermia, heat rash, lowered immunity, suicide, constipation…'

Derek thrust out his jaw and looked impassive. He was already beginning to look like a proletarian hero.

'Ooh, what's this one?' said Angie. 'Ooh yucky!'

'What?' asked Derek suspiciously.

'Eeugh!' said Angie.

'What?' demanded Derek.

'You'll get something called lanugo. When hairs grow all over your body.'

'All over his body?' asked Jasmine.

'Yes.'

'Ooh yuck!' said Jasmine.

'Not ordinary hairs either,' continued Angie. 'They're a special sort of hair. That's why they're called lanugo.'

'What do they look like?' asked Derek uneasily.

'It doesn't say.'

'Probably a bit like noodles,' suggested Stuart.

'Yuck!' repeated Jasmine, looking more and more disgusted.

'You didn't tell me that, Pete,' said Derek irritably.

'Lanugo *doesn't* look like noodles,' I explained. 'It looks fine. There's nothing wrong with it either. Babies sometimes have it, and elephants, and anyway …,' but Derek wasn't listening.

'All over your body?' he repeated.

'Yes,' said Angie.

'Not like normal hair?'

'No.'

Derek thought for a moment. Then he looked at his watch.

'Well,' he said, 'I've tried it for a bit and I think that's about long enough.'

Then he ate another biscuit.

The Revolutionary Diet in Three Nutshells

Join a cell
Make things in a shed
Eat nothing at all

Sources

M. Ende, *The Grey Gentlemen*
K. Marx, and F. Engels *The Communist Manifesto*
K. Marx, The Economic and Philosophical Manuscripts of 1844
K. Marx, *The Eighteenth Brumaire*
Plato, *The Republic*

Dear Edna
How nice that things are back to normal again! I know that you are very busy with the young mums group just now, so under the circumstances we were most grateful for the chocolate biscuits. They were very tasty, although they were just a tiny bit over cooked. Next time could they be a little bit more 'doughy'?

Yours ever,
Peter

Chapter 6
Hegel's Dialectical Diet

which explains how in order to become slim it first necessary to be fat.

GWF Hegel cutting his hair

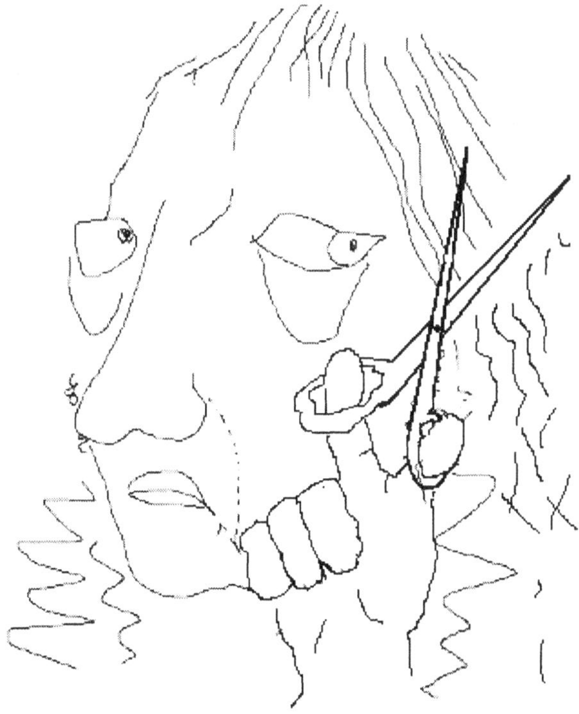

Hegel uses very complicated language. Indeed it is so complicated that very few people are intelligent enough to understand what on earth he is talking about (luckily I happen to be one of them). For example, I bet you cannot work out what this means:

> The genus ... is present in the individual as a straining against the inadequacy of its single actuality, as the urge to obtain its self-feeling in the other of its genus, to integrate itself through union with it and through the mediation to close the genus with itself and bring it into existence.*

But underneath all this complexity there is a simple idea. Everything in the world, in fact in the whole universe, is changing, and these changes occur in three stages: (1) the thesis, (2) the antithesis, (3) the synthesis. The thesis comes first then, somehow, it manages to create its very opposite which is the antithesis. Because the thesis and the antithesis are opposites, they will have some sort of battle with each other. Sometimes this is just an argument; sometimes it is literally a fight or a war. Out of this battle emerges the synthesis, which is a mixture of the two. This is called the 'Hegelian Dialectic.' For example (and this will be important for our diet), according to Hegel men and women are not basically the same, in fact they are better described as opposites: man is the thesis, woman the antithesis. When they come together to have a child, the child provides a synthesis, one that draws man and woman together in a family. The family in turn becomes the thesis; in a family everyone loves one another and has a strong sense of their duty to support and help each other. Many families create a society, which is the antithesis of family life because people in society are selfish

---

*G.W.F. Hegel, *Philosophy of Nature*, para. 368, tr. A.V. Miller, Oxford, 1970. It means wanting to have sex.

and calculating to each other and want to cheat others rather than help them. The synthesis is the state that draws the family and society together. What kind of state might this be? Well, first the king—who appears like God—makes all the law, so he is the thesis. But the idea that a god-like king can lay down whatever law he likes creates an antithesis in rebels who say that the king is just an ordinary human being like everyone else, so they can ignore the law. Tyranny (thesis) creates anarchy (antithesis), until eventually a synthesis emerges in a democratic form of government with law based on a constitution.

The Hegelian Dialectic

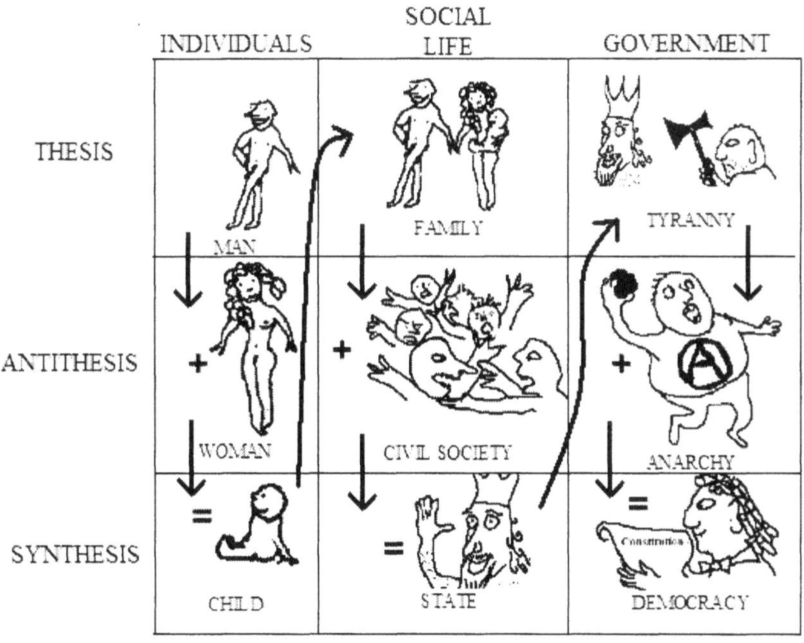

Once you start to get the idea, you begin to notice that you can see thesis-antithesis-synthesis everywhere. For example, the story of Goldilocks and the three bears is Hegelian dialectics through and through: the thesis is father bear's porridge, the antithesis is mother bear's porridge, the synthesis is baby bear's porridge, and so on.

It will not take you long for you to work out that when it comes to losing weight, the same basic pattern turns up in what we can call the Dieting Dialectic:

Step one (the thesis) is being too thin
Step two (the antithesis) is being too fat
Step three (the synthesis) is being just right

The dieting dialectic, therefore, says that before you can reach the final ideal of being slim (but not thin) you must first be fat.

'But,' I hear you say, 'I don't *want* to get fat first.'

That is all right. You already *are* fat. What you need to do, of course, is to move from the antithesis (being overweight), to the synthesis (being the right weight). Easy to say! The question is how to get there. Now Hegel provides a fascinating answer, and when all is said and done, one that is surprisingly easy to understand.

The Diet Dialectic

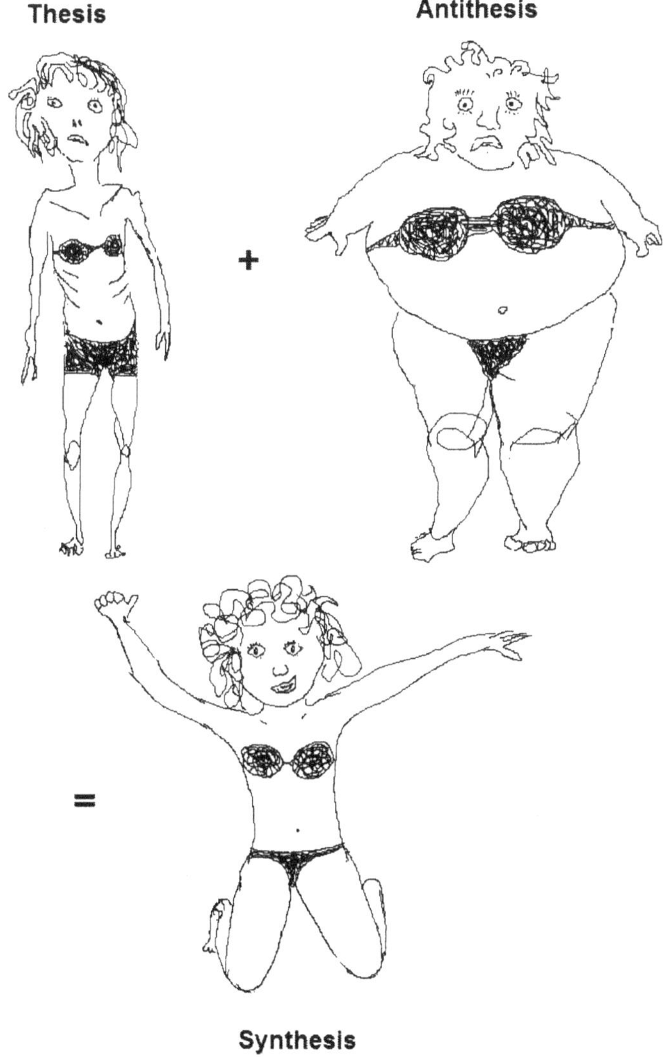

Dieting and Happiness

Do you remember John Locke reversing cause and effect in his analysis of our metabolism? Well, Hegel reverses cause and effect too, and in an amazing mind-body way.

Here is the usual argument, one that you are all familiar with. Ask yourself if you agree or disagree with this statement:

Being overweight causes me to be unhappy.

Often true? True of yourself? Well, Hegel says not that it is false exactly, but rather that it is *backwards*. What is really going on is this:

Being unhappy causes me to be overweight.

If Hegel is right this is fantastic news for anyone who is concerned at being overweight. It means that if we want to lose weight there is no need to spend our time counting the calories, no need even to spend it sitting on a bucket. To lose weight *all you have to do is be happy!* Provided that you can hit on some way to be truly deeply happy, then you will *effortlessly* and *spontaneously* start shedding fat.

Why would Hegel make such an astonishing claim, and why should we believe him? To understand why Hegel thinks happiness makes us lose weight, we need to understand two things about his philosophy, beginning with the unhappy consciousness.

The Unhappy Consciousness

When Hegel started to work on his philosophical ideas he was not thinking about the problem of how to go on a diet. Rather, he wanted to know why we human beings have made progress. Why have we had any history at all? Why, for example, are we not still living rather like a bear, sleeping in caves and eating raw food? Or if you want to take things forward a bit, why do we not still live in the village Plato described in his diet of pigs, following a simple life singing and going around naked? Hegel's answer is that when we lived like this, *it made someone unhappy*. And because they were unhappy they decided to do something to *change* it. To change things the unhappy person found they had to change *the whole way of life in their community*, usually by fighting a war. Hegel calls such people World Historical Individuals. Alexander the Great was one, and Julius Caesar, and Napoleon. More recently the great human rights campaigner Martin Luther King would fit the pattern. There was racism; he was unhappy about it; he acted, and the world changed.

It is interesting to ask yourself who else might be a world historical individual, provided you realise that there are not very many of them.* For example, you cannot say, 'I think my schoolteacher is a world historical individual because they inspired me to do my best.' Schoolteachers do not count, they are just *ordinary*. In fact, almost all human beings are just ordinary. Instead of going round killing people like Alexander the Great did they do ordinary things. And instead

* Diet 'gurus' often pose as world historical individuals. They claim to have some great new 'secret' idea, and promise to lead their unhappy and overweight flock to becoming slim and happy. We know they are fake because the population of the world just keeps getting fatter.

of feeling intensely passionate about what they are doing, they have ordinary feelings. So what do ordinary people do when they are unhappy? Do they find themselves gripped by a burning desire to go out and change the society they live in, or even the whole world? No they don't. They just grow fat.

One of the more unpleasant things about Hegel is that he does not seem to care very much about ordinary people being unhappy, and hence fat. In fact, it may be worse even than that. The more people who are unhappy, the more likely it is that *one* of them will turn into a world historical individual that achieves some kind of progress. If everyone was happy, then the human race would never achieve anything. It is only because one or two exceptional people are unhappy that history moves forward. The problem is that you cannot know in advance who these amazing people are going to be, so the more people who are unhappy the better. Finding this extraordinary individual is a bit like finding a pearl in a bed of wild oysters. Just as you have to cut open thousands of oysters to find the pearl, so you have to make thousands or millions of people unhappy to create a world historical individual. If the only way that everyone else can cope with unhappiness is by becoming overweight, that is just their hard luck.

So Hegel positively *wants* people to be unhappy, and if that makes them fat, he couldn't care less. This helps to explain why his solution to how to lose weight and look great is hidden in a cunning metaphor deep inside his philosophy. Indeed, this metaphor has been so cunningly hidden, that it is almost completely unknown, so that it is only now that I can reveal Hegel's secret to you.

The Secret of Spontaneous Generation

What happens, Hegel asks, when we eat so much that we become full to bursting? His answer is that a tapeworm grows in our stomach. Hegel stresses that being afflicted with tapeworm is emphatically *not* the result of inadvertently swallowing its eggs or anything like that, rather it is created *directly* as a result of our over eating. In other words, eating too much means that a tapeworm is *spontaneously generated* inside us.

Hegelian scholars have maintained a conspiracy of silence over this illuminating passage, perhaps because they cannot understand why on earth Hegel believed in spontaneous generation when—as any educated person would know—it had been decisively disproved by Francesco Redi more than a hundred years earlier. There are, however, two possible explanations. The first is that Hegel's belief in spontaneous generation fits neatly into the idea of the thesis creating the antithesis. In this case eating too much is the thesis which creates the antithesis of a tapeworm eating the food inside you. But if this explanation is true, if Hegel really believes that regardless of the evidence tapeworms appear as if by magic just because his theory of dialectics demands it, then it raises the distinct possibility that the rest of his philosophy might be equally silly. No wonder Hegelians tend not to talk about it.

But there is a second and I believe much better explanation for what Hegel means in this mysterious secret passage. Hegel did not literally believe that a tapeworm would appear spontaneously. Rather he was using the tapeworm as a *metaphor.* Now a tapeworm actually provides a way of losing weight, because instead of your food turning into fat, the tapeworm eats it. With this in mind, Hegel's metaphor was this: The very fact that you are fat creates inside you something that can make you slim. You are fat because you are unhappy. This means that you have dormant inside you the antithesis of being fat; you have an inner tapeworm of happiness. If you can just wake up that happy tapeworm, it will eat away all your excess weight. Metaphorically then, we do not want to get rid of our tapeworm. In fact, a tapeworm is exactly what we *need*.

Inner Happiness

As soon as I explained it to them, the Guinea Pigs loved the metaphor of the happy tapeworm. Stuart was especially enthusiastic. As things transpired he did not actually understand what the word 'metaphor' meant, and had slightly missed the point. Some of the subsequent misunderstandings have (as usual) been blamed on me, but in my defence he apparently comprehended the matter perfectly well. Indeed, I remember that he *said* he understood after Jasmine had confessed that she did not. Jasmine had sighed, looked downcast, and said:

'Sorry, I know it's going to hold us up, but I'm not sure I can get this tapeworm thing. I mean where…'

And Stuart had butted in:

'Well, *I* can get it. It's easy,'

Then, in what I naturally took at the time to be a further metaphor (although actually it was not), Stuart announced that he and Wendy were going on another holiday, this time to the tropics, where he would feast on some local culinary speciality—though the guidebooks said not to. Wendy quickly butted in to add that she was sorry that this time I could not come. She was not saying that I had ruined their last trip, but all in all she and Stuart thought that this time they would rather go on their own.

A holiday, taken in the right spirit, can be a lasting source of happiness. Many years ago on a backpacking trip I met a young man on a Cretan beach. It was very wild and remote and he had been there since the winter, sleeping in a cave, watching the storms, all alone. But now the summer was coming and the beach began to fill up as people clambered down from the winding goat paths to pitch their tents or lie beneath the stars, drinking from the pure spring water that welled up from beneath the cliff. By a curious fluke the new occupants of the beach were almost entirely made up of beautiful naked women. These he austerely ignored, but they had a wasp-and-jam pot effect, and soon out of nowhere speedboats were landing and then someone arrived and built a wooden bar at one end of the bay. It was this that finally drove the young man away. He was philosophical about the destruction of his idyll when I met him again, by chance, on the ferry back to Athens. 'I hope that some of the peace that I found there will remain inside me when I get back to Germany.' He was, of course, German, and I think that he was also happy with a kind of happiness goes deeper than sitting in front of a movie with a bag of popcorn. Needless to add, although he was entirely unconscious of his appearance, he looked great and had an iron stomach.

The Happiness Ceremony

Hegel thinks that special events and 'magic' rituals are really important, because they get people to commit to things. So for the benefit of the Guinea Pigs and to get the message across that Hegel's secret to losing weight and looking great is inner happiness I combined a ceremony with a conjuring trick. If you are going to follow the dieting dialectic, you will want to do something similar.

(1) I got out a piggy back.

(2) I passed round some small sheets of paper, and asked everyone to write their name, and in a few words, something that would make *them* happy.

'There is no right or wrong answer,' I said. 'Just write down what you feel.'

(3) Once everyone had written down what would make them happy, I asked them to fold it up and put it through the piggy bank slot.

Everyone did as I asked except Derek who looked at me suspiciously and then folded his written piece of paper tightly and put it into his shirt pocket. I let it pass.

'This piggy bank is *you'* I said, 'and the secret of inner happiness is already inside you, just like those slips of paper are inside the pig. Now you just need to *find* that happiness.'

I put the piggy bank in a cardboard box and closed the lid.

'Everyone put their hand on the box,' I said. They all did (Derek put his hand to his pocket).

'Now repeat after me: "I promise to follow my dream of inner happiness".'

They all promised.

If you keep that promise and obtain inner happiness,' I said, 'it will *change* the outer you.' Then I opened the cardboard box.

The Guinea Pigs all gasped in amazement.* The piggybank had vanished. In its place was a Barbie Doll.

'OK, I said, 'now go away and chase after that dream!'

---

* Except Derek.

After the Guinea Pigs had gone, I got the piggy bank out from where I had hidden it under the table and opened it up. This is what I read:

Wendy: 'Stuart to lose weight'
Stuart: 'Wendy to be like she used to be again'
Angie: 'Promotion at work'
Jasmine: 'A nice haircut'

As I had expected, Wendy and Stuart were locked into what Hegel calls a master-slave dialectic with Wendy as the master and Stuart as the slave. Until we got on to Nietzsche's überdiet, there was nothing much I could do about this, it would just have to run its course. As for the others, Jasmine had got the answer right, and Angie had got the answer wrong.

I had given the Guinea Pigs Hegel's advice that if you want to lose weight and look great you should be happy. What I had not yet mentioned to them was that Hegel's route to happiness was, in part, to act in accordance with the characteristics of your sex. In other words, if you are a man you should be masculine, and if you are a women you should be feminine. Angie's mistake was to see happiness in terms of masculine striving. Only Jasmine, with her decidedly feminine interest in hair care, was in tune with the happiness-needs of her sex, and I felt that with a bit of extra tuition, the dieting dialectic could be really helpful to her.

Sex and the Animal-Vegetable Antithesis

As we now live in a democracy we would think that we ought to be happy, and if happy, then slim. But as we have seen, people in democratic countries tend to be overweight, and thanks to Hegel we now know that they are overweight because they are unhappy. So what has gone wrong with democracy? Hegel's answer is that democracy has its own thesis-antithesis-synthesis sequence. (1) The thesis is that men and women are *different* and *unequal*: men are seen as superior to women and boss them around. A society where men lord it over women around will have all kind of other vicious hierarchies too, with the result that most of the population, whatever their sex, will be ill fed through poverty, and rather thin. (2) The antithesis is the belief that men and women are *equal* because they are *the same*. This is the modern reality as women gain all kinds of opportunities in business, the professions and in public life. They compete with men on equal terms, and often outperform them. We have women prime ministers, women doctors, women millionaires and women boxing at the Olympics. Meanwhile, more and more men stay at home, cooking, cleaning and looking after the children. That, Hegel says, makes both men and women unhappy (and hence overweight) because actually they are *not* the same. (3) The synthesis is the realisation that men and women are *equal*, but they are also *different*. If you can achieve this synthesis you will become happy—and lose weight!

Let's be clear, Hegel is sexist. But perhaps, just possibly, Hegel is *right* to be sexist. We have seen how ever since Plato it has been known that democracy makes us overweight. Could it also be that our current ideas of sex-equality have also contributed to the obesity epidemic? And if you are offended by Hegel's idea that the achievement of women's rights has made people fat, then all I can say is *what did you expect*? I told you that these philosophers were not very nice.

Hegel put the difference between the sexes like this:

Men are like animals women are like plants.

What did he mean? The obvious difference between an animal and a plant is that an animal moves around and a plant stays in one place. Well, for Hegel men move around and women stay put. It is the men who go out doing things, it is the women who stay at home. Men drive forward politics and business, while women tend to domestic matters. Men look outwards to change the world, women think only of their family. So a man satisfies himself by *doing* things, and a woman satisfies herself just by *being* a woman. This means that men and woman are not just different, they are opposites, just as animals and vegetables are opposite life forms.

The Dialectic of Equality

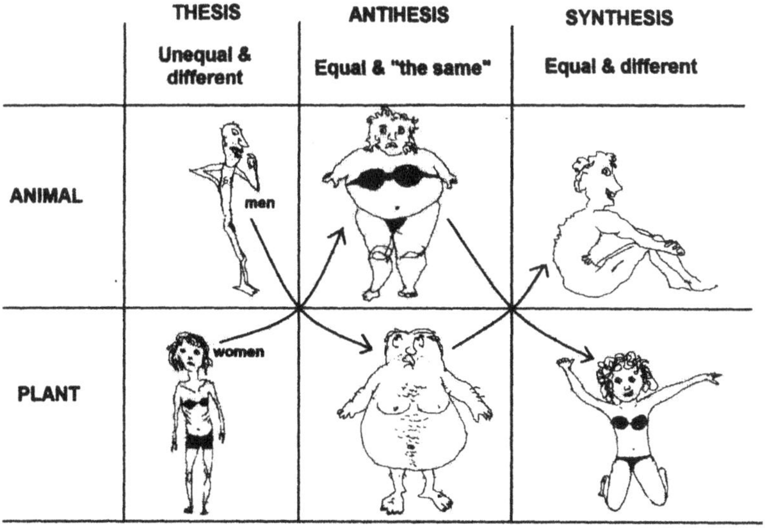

	THESIS Unequal & different	ANTIHESIS Equal & "the same"	SYNTHESIS Equal & different
ANIMAL	men		
PLANT	women		

OK. Imagine Hegel knocks on the door. You are surprised; you were not expecting Hegel and in fact assumed it would be someone else, but of course you invite him in. He is here to explain why men are like animals and women are like plants. He sketches out a diagram of boxes and arrows that shows how, as men and women become equal, women become more like animals, men more like plants, and both become fat. He explains that to be slim, overweight people need to realise that being equal does not mean being the same. Then he asks an intriguing question:

'Do you have a pet? A dog, a cat, a tortoise?*

'Yes? Good! Bring your pet over here so that it can sit on your lap. Now, I want you to notice something that is different between you and your pet: you are much more expressive than it is. You have a face that shows if you are happy or sad. In fact, your face can show a whole range of thoughts and feelings. Compare that with your cat (or whatever). It is very difficult to tell from its face anything about its inner emotional state. True, you might be able to work out a few things: If a tortoise hides in its shell it is frightened. If a dog wags its tail it is happy. But compared to the range of expression of a human being, there is not much that an animal can tell you. The inner you, your emotions, your desires are shown on the surface far more than anything that is revealed by your pet.

'Now,' Hegel continues, 'I would like you to pull up your top so that we can look at your stomach. I am a doctor of philosophy so there is no need to be embarrassed. That's right.

* In fact almost any pet will do. The only real exceptions are some of the more translucent varieties of tropical fish.

Yes. Good. OK. What I want you to notice is how when you compare your skin with the fur (or the shell) of your pet, the skin is much more revealing. All that fur covers up the inner animal, and this makes its posture and feelings much more hard to see. But your exposed skin is rather like your face in showing something about what you are feeling. Of course it does not show everything, I cannot see you internal organs for example, but what I can see is still telling of your inner being. If your muscles are straining with effort, it shows through your skin. If your heart is palpitating, I can see this too. If—as you are at the moment—you are blushing, this is also evident on your skin.

'But the problem,' says Hegel gesturing to your stomach, 'is all this fat. It hides the inner you, rather like the fur of an animal. If you were a man it would hide the straining of your muscles 'Of course in your case,' Hegel would continue, 'I know you are a woman.' (I should mention at this point that 'Hegel' is actually me and that I am talking to Jasmine, who has a cat.) 'To be a beautiful women is to reveal your inner nature: one that is shown in the soft graceful curves of your body beneath your skin. Because women are plant-like and still, their beauty is shaped by fat not muscle. They are beautiful just by being there.' (Male beauty, by contrast, is muscular because it is associated with activity, with struggling to do something.)

'When women get too fat they lose their beautiful curves. The fat becomes like an animal's fur. It conceals the inner woman, rather than expresses it. So a fat woman is rather like a furry pet, covering up their inner being. To lose weight is to get rid of all that furry animal fat, to show their plant like beauty inside. I am sure you have heard the joke that inside every fat person there is a thin person struggling to get out. Well, inside every overweight woman, there is a beautiful woman struggling to reveal herself.'

Suspicions of Derek

At this point, 'Hegel,' who as I have mentioned was really me, paused for breath and Jasmine asked if she could pull her top down again. We were in Jasmine's flat so I was totally shocked when a moment later Derek came bursting in through the door with a paintbrush and a takeaway Indian meal. He seemed equally surprised to see me. Had I come round to help with the painting too? Most certainly not.

'He's been feeling my stomach' interjected Jasmine.

'All part of the diet dialectic' I added quickly.

Derek did not like this, and started to quiz me.

'If it is part of the dieting club, then why aren't you filming it?' he asked. (I was still pretending to the GPs that we were making a documentary.)

'As a matter of fact I *am* filming it,' I replied, pointing to the camcorder.

But this did not seem to make things any better, and instead of apologising Derek put the most perverse interpretation on our private consultation. We had a bit of an argument, and I thought it best to leave.

Derek's suspicions were, of course, entirely unfounded; I had acted with the most scrupulous professionalism throughout and I mention the incident at all only because it sowed an ugly and malevolent seed in Derek's mind. I was able to rise above our little contretemps. Derek let it fester.

Suspicions of Angie

We were back in the church hall. At least Angie and I were. Stuart and Wendy were on holiday and Derek and Jasmine had not turned up.

'I heard all about it from Jasmine,' said Angie. 'Pete, what *were* you doing?'

'Nothing, honestly, look I'll show you.'

I tried to demonstrate but I may as well admit that the philosophical detachment that I had maintained in prodding Jasmine's stomach soon vanished when it came to Angie. Angie was definitely 'my type'—articulate, intelligent, sometimes fiery and impulsive, but also thoughtful and kind. And Hegel was right. Trying to feel beneath Angie's fat by poking around her midriff made feel that I was getting closer to those most attractive qualities. So things 'began to happen', but there is no need to draw a veil over what, because they had hardly got very far when there was a knock at the door.

'Just ignore it Angie.'

'After what kicked off last time? You're joking!'

'It's only the Vicar's wife and she can leave the tray outside'.

'Yes she *could*, but what if she opens the door?' said Angie pushing my hand away and pulling down her top. 'Come in Edna!'

Instead of the Vicar's wife it was the Vicar. He marched into the room angrily brandishing a fist full of letters. They were the thank you notes I had sent to his spouse.

'What do you mean by these?'

'They're just friendly little notes.'

'Well you can stop it. And don't pretend that you believe all the things about forgiveness and love, you're just saying them so she makes you more cakes.'

I pondered a dialectical response to this accusation, but as it was, in fact, true, I decided to hold my peace. The Vicar however, had plenty more to say. On the very first session, he complained, we had left brown stains on the floor. (Here I could reassure him that these were only the remains of his wife's chocolate cake.) Not only that, but I had written 'Religion is the opium of the people' on the whiteboard, not the sort of thing that he wanted the young mums to read. (This was not deliberate, I had been explaining Marx's attitude to dieting and had simply forgotten to wipe it off.) Finally:

'You made the most disgusting mess in the toilet the other week too, and my wife had to clean it up.'

I had been patient until then, but this was the last straw.

'With all the vast resources of the Church of England at your disposal you force your wife to clean toilets?' You treat your wife like a slave! Censoring her correspondence, denying her the feminine happiness of baking cakes. You're not so much a vicar as a tyrant!'

This caused another argument. The Vicar became noisy and aggressive, as was his wont, while I explained how in his attitude to marriage he was stuck at the 'thesis' stage of Hegel's dialectic of equality. I was rather pleased at how I had turned his entrance to pedagogical advantage for understanding Hegelianism, and was hoping that Angie had noticed. But she was absorbed in reading the notes, and after the Vicar had left she showed no inclination to resume our stomach prodding.

'You know it *was* a bit funny, you turning up in Jasmine's flat, she mused, 'and now you've been writing these letters to Edna too.'

'I know, I was such an idiot complaining about them being overcooked because obviously now she's taken offence.

But some of them were actually *burnt*, I mean if no one mentions it, how are you ever going to know?'

'I wasn't talking about Edna's cookies,' said Angie sharply. 'I'm kind of thinking Peter, what are you about? Am I just another woman for you to play with?'

'No Angie, of course not. I mean I went round to Jasmine's to feel her stomach, yes. But with Jasmine, she can't think things through like you can, she can't discuss things, argue things. In fact she can't really do any of the things I really like about you. The thing was that for this diet her *instincts* were right. Jasmine's wish was for a new hairstyle, and that meant she wanted to nurture herself like a plant, to be more womanly. *That's* why I went round. I really thought Hegel's diet might suit her.'

'You mean like a man might try to become more manly by shaving all his hair off so that he looks like a soldier or a thug? But because I'm a woman I should grow my hair long and spend my time washing and combing it and arranging it beautifully?'

'Exactly. Hair growth is rather like plant growth so feminine women should cultivate their hair, while men should keep it short.* Incidentally, that's why Hegel is the only great German thinker who is not conspicuously hairy.'

'And what about my wish, how was *my* instinct?'

'Ah. Yes, promotion at work. No, that was no good. That was masculine ambition; it won't make you happy and lose weight, it'll only make the problem worse.'

---

* Hegel thinks that hairy men, far from exhibiting an animalistic vitality, are actually showing a vegetable-like weakness. He gets this idea from Johann Wolfgang von Goethe.

Angie snorted. 'You said that there were world historical individuals? Well, we women have our *own* world historical individuals, like the suffragettes, that woman who got trodden on by a horse, the Pankhursts. They gave us the idea of being equal to men and you can't put the genie back in the bottle. We want to be free, we want to get out there and do things like men, and you are saying we should move backwards and be decorative household objects! What rubbish. If that's Hegel's philosophy, he's a male chauvinist pig!'

'In a way, Angie you're right. Look, Hegel certainly wants women to be free (that's the thesis). But Hegel also wants women to be feminine rather than masculine, which means doing traditional womanly things (that's the antithesis). So how do you square that circle? If you are a woman, you have to *freely choose* to be feminine (the synthesis). You have to decide to squeeze yourself back in that feminine bottle. But do not think of it as a bottle. Think of it instead as a beautifully shaped hourglass.'

'Is that so?' said Angie in a rather unpleasant tone of voice. 'We women have to give up all we have achieved in the last two hundred years and go back to being what Hegel calls "plants?" '

'If you want to be happy and slim: Yes.'

'For a woman, that is the most insulting so-called philosophy of dieting I have ever heard. No, you can't stroke my stomach any more, keep your dirty paws off. I'm leaving.'

'It's not *my* idea Angie, it's Hegel.' But Angie wasn't staying to listen, she slammed the door and left. After the intimacy of our stomach prodding session this was frustrating in the short term, but in the long term felt I could afford to be philosophical. To achieve a really satisfactory synthesis with

Angie it was good to have some antithetical conflict with her first. She would be back for Schopenhauer. But—I mused—if she though *Hegel* was bad .... I thought of Schopenhauer's 'Essay on Women' which, even by his standards, was rather blunt. How could I possibly explain *that* to Angie? Dialectically of course, that went without saying, but how?

The Dieting Dialectic in a Nutshell

1. Become happy and so lose weight.
2. Perform a Happiness Ceremony:

(a) Write down things that will make you happy and more feminine (if a woman), or masculine (if a man).
(b)Put the list in a piggy bank. Put your hand on it and promise to do what it says. Make the piggy bank 'vanish' and replace it with the new you as a slim doll. (Men can use an 'action man' or similar figure.)

Sources

J. Conrad, *Under Western Eyes*
GWF Hegel, *Aesthetics*
GWF Hegel, *Philosophy of Nature*
GWF Hegel, *Philosophy of Right*
GWF Hegel, *Reason in History*

Chapter 7
Schopenhauer's Women's Diet

which explains how your imagination can help you to lose weight.

Arthur Schopenhauer philosophises on women

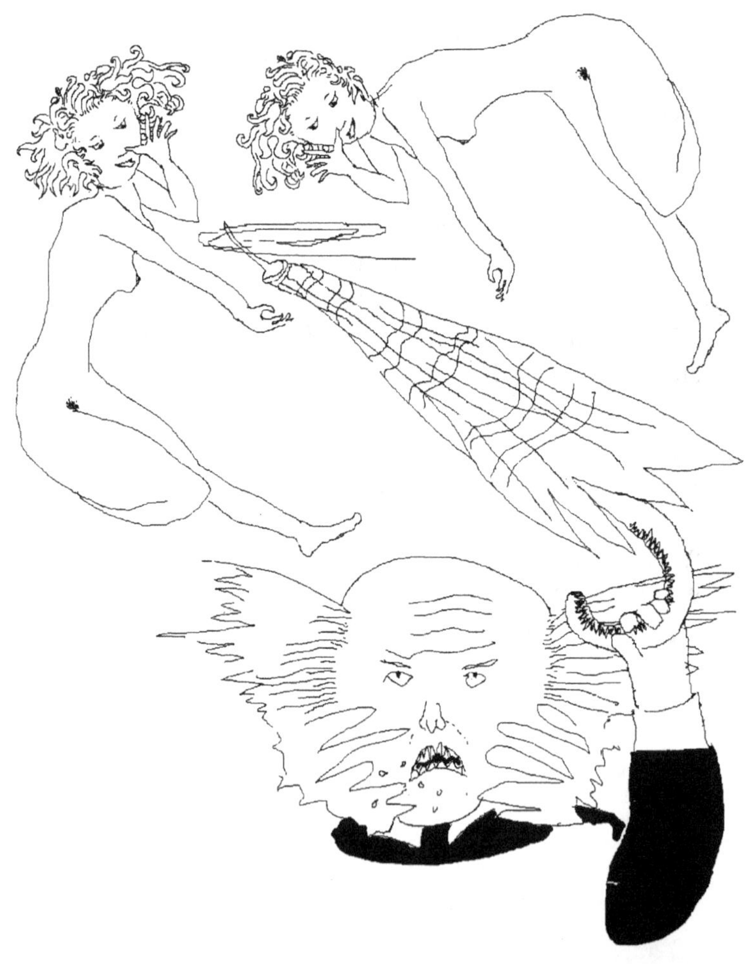

Oddly enough it was Stuart infecting himself with tapeworms while on holiday that gave me the idea of how to explain Schopenhauer. While other guests cowered inside the compound of their luxury hotel, Stuart had swaggered out into the local markets living dangerously by eating various undercooked meat dishes. The results were all too predictable and he was now receiving hospital treatment. Wendy, who told me about Stuart's illness, added rather shortly that neither of them would be attending any more diet meetings. But every cloud has its silver lining, and Stuart's inability to understand that Hegel's passage on the spontaneous generation of intestinal parasites was a metaphor, was to prove invaluable in getting across the message of one of the most difficult of the nineteenth century German philosophers.

The rest of us, Angela, Jasmine, Derek, and I were back in the church hall. But the atmosphere was tense: the conflicts that had been generated by the Hegelian dialectic had left some raw feelings. We all needed to relax, calm down and reconnect with each other, so I brewed some tea and handed round a packet of biscuits, which for obvious reasons were from the supermarket.

'I am going to tell you a story,' I said, 'one that I want you to remember every time you look in a mirror. And to help you remember it, I've got a little picture of a sort of crab parasite, called a sacculina that I want you to stick on your fridge when you get home.'

I gave everyone in the Guinea Pig Gang a picture as shown.

Fridge Picture

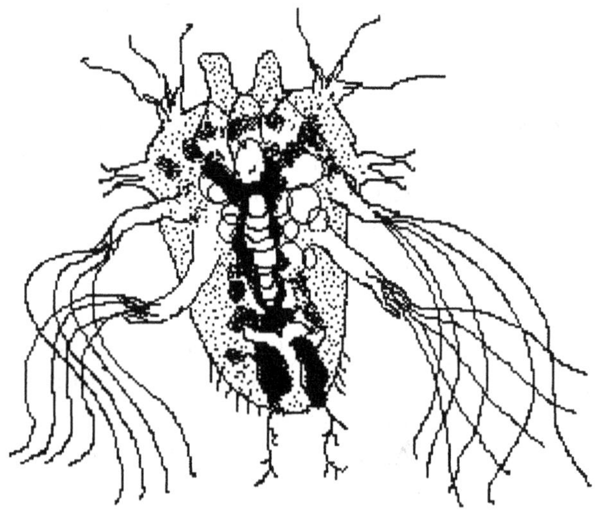

Sacculina carcini

You, the reader, will need a similar picture for *your* fridge. You can copy this one, or draw your own, or download an image from the internet.

'In this story,' I told the three remaining members of the gang, '*you* are the heroine or the hero. And what I want you to do two things. First, while I am telling you the story, I want you to imagine, as hard as you can, that the story is *true*. But then, at the end of the story, I'm going to ask you to imagine something else as hard as you can: I want you to imagine that the story is *false*.'

Angie and Jasmine were willing to give it a try, so I asked them to relax, close their eyes, hold their stomachs and listen. Derek, however, merely rolled his eyes, picked up a magazine that Jasmine had brought and started to study the swimsuit photos.

I ignored Derek and concentrated on the other two, and this is what I said:

Somewhere in the tropics is a banana republic. It is a beautiful country, green and lush, inhabited by a beautiful, lithe and graceful people. This is where you live. And you, at the start of this story, you are beautiful too, at least, you have a superb body: no spare fat, looking just as nature intended. Beautiful in youth, dignified in age. And age too carries with it its own beauty.

The country should be a happy place. But it is not, because it is ruled by a brutal dictator.

El Presidenté.

El Presidenté is evil and sadistic and the people live in fear of his tyranny with its secret police and its torture chambers.

There is only one person who is brave enough to challenge his vile regime.

You.

You speak out against El Presidenté. You make a speech. It is a courageous speech in which you demand justice and freedom and human rights for all. You are heroic to have done this, because you know the consequences.

When El Presidenté hears what you have said he is furious. He howls with rage, and when he finally calms down it is only to send out his goons to arrest you and bring you back to his palace, where he plans to throw you into a bath of acid. That's what he usually does to those who cross him. But while he is waiting for the bath to fill, his CIA minder comes in and pulls the plug.

'You can't do that El Presidenté, not this time.'

El Presidenté snorts angrily and his frothing lips twist into an ugly sneer.

'Whaddaya mean I can't do it? I can do whatever I damn well like.'

'This Mandela wannabe' (that is what the CIA man calls you), 'their speech is all over the TV. If you liquidate them, Sir, Congress might kick up.' (This story is set in the bad old days when America occasionally supported dictatorships so that its multinational companies could steal a country's land and exploit its people.)

'So what? A bit of fuss, it dies down...'

'They might withdraw you freedom medal,' says the CIA man who, for reasons of his own, is anxious to keep you in one piece.

El Presidenté instinctively puts his hand to his chest where his Congressional Medal of Freedom glistens. The CIA man glances at him shrewdly.

'I could buy another one,' says El Presidenté, I bought a Victoria Cross once.'

'Sure you could *buy* one, Sir, but buying it doesn't count. And that's not all Mr President. There's a lot of pinkos in Congress these days. ('Pinkos' was the CIA man's name for Members of Congress who supported human rights.) You go kill this human rights big mouth and they just might stop sending you your annual One Billion Dollars in Humanitarian Aid.'

'Well what am I gona do then?' El Presidenté snarls in frustration. 'You want me to do nothing and let this commie terrorist' (that is what he calls you) 'get away with it?'

'No Sir,' says the CIA man. 'We want you to do something all right. Fact is Mr President, we've got something new to try, something the biotech boys have just put together.'

The CIA man opens the lid of his briefcase, pulls out a simple looking television remote control box, shuts the briefcase again quickly, and hands the control box to El Presidenté.

'This is for you, Sir.'

El Presidenté looks at the control box. It has three buttons, a big red one in the middle, and two smaller ones labelled 'manual' and 'automatic.'

'What's this?' asks El Presidenté pressing the red button.

There is a sudden scrabbling sound inside the briefcase.

'Whoa! Not yet!' says the CIA man anxiously. 'OK let's wait until the thing calms down.'

'What calms down?'

'You'll see in a moment Sir.'

Slowly and cautiously the CIA man opens the briefcase. There, squatting inside is a small black tubular looking thing with long legs, or perhaps wires. It is not clear if it is an animal or a machine. It resembles a spider or an octopus, but it also looks like a tiny radio with branching antennae. El Presidenté peers at it curiously. Suddenly it scrabbles again.

The CIA man slams down the lid while El Presidenté, who like all bullies is a coward at heart, jumps back, crosses himself and blasphemes.

'Holy Motherfucker of God! What *was* that thing?'

'The lab boys call it 'the Fat Widow' because it looks a bit like a spider and it loves food. It probably smelt something on your breath just then.'

'What we gona do with it?'

'Get Big Mouth Mandela to swallow it,' says the CIA man, winking at the President.

El Presidenté's face assumes a nasty leer.

'Yeah? Tell me more *amigo*, sounds like that could be fun.'

'Fun, Sir?' The CIA allows himself the smallest flicker of a smile. 'The fun start *afterwards*.'

***

An hour later you are hustled into the presidential palace and thrust into a room. The room has been fashioned, in accordance with one of El Presidenté's little whims, to look like a Cotswold cottage. There are wooden beams on the ceiling with a row of horse brasses nailed to them. A slightly curious looking camera that is also attached to the beams is pointing at you. There is a painting of a Constable landscape on the wall, a table, a blue checked teacloth, a set of willow pattern china, a jar of jam, a plate of scones and a bowl of clotted cream. El Presidenté himself is sat at the table fingering his remote control box and the CIA man is standing in the corner with his briefcase, his face impassive.

'Do sit down,' says El Presidenté,' with fake politeness.

You sit and El Presidenté pours tea.

'I heard that speech,' says El Presidenté, 'and you make me sound like I'm some kind of pig. But you got it all wrong. I'm civilised. And to prove it, we gona have a tea and scones just like in jolly old England. Here, take a scone.'

'No, thank you,' you reply with dignity.

'OK, I'll eat it then.' El Presidenté takes back the scone he had offered, dips it in the jam, smears it with clotted cream and stuffs it into his mouth, covering his face in cream and crumbs.

The man in the corner coughs and makes a gesture of wiping his finger round the corner of his lips. El Presidenté takes the hint; he swallows the last of the scone and meticulously wipes his mouth clean on the tablecloth. Then he slurps his tea spits on the floor and offers you the plate.

'Go on, take one. You have to eat sometime or you gona starve to death.'

You take a scone. You put it close to your mouth, and sniff. It smells fine. But then why is El Presidenté eying you so intently with his malevolent piggy eyes?

'You see. Like I said. Civilised: the Queen, Winston Churchill and all that.'

You open your mouth and start to take a bite.

All of a sudden the man in the corner opens his briefcase and something small and black with long legs flies out. It skittles across the room up your legs and body and into your mouth. A moment later and it has forced itself down your throat.

'Eugh! What?'

'Well well well. You swallowed a fly!' jokes El Presidenté. Then he starts laughing a foul hyena-like laugh, while the man with the briefcase sidles out of the corner.

'Actually, you've just swallowed a most remarkable piece of biotechnology Miss Mandela.'

You conceal your fright at what has happened and answer him quietly. 'That's not my name.'

'I'm so sorry. Mrs Mandela? Mr Mandela? Whatever. Anyway, you'll be wanting to know the name of the thing that's now in your stomach. So I'll tell you. Its official name is an autosacculina, but we'll just call it the Fat Widow. Stay there a minute and we'll see where it's got to.'

The camera on the ceiling flashes, the Constable painting on the wall disappears behind a white screen, and a gently pulsating black and white image appears.

'That's your stomach in ultrasound, and you can just make out the Fat Widow ... there.' The man points at a dark spot on the screen. 'You see the filaments, the lines emanating out from it? Those are its arms. Some of them are feeling their way up past your lungs through your shoulders and into *your* arms. These other ones are rooting their way down to your legs. This one here' – he points – 'is climbing back up into your throat. When it gets to the uvula it will divide and spread into your jaws and your tongue. In fact, in a minute or two the Fat Widow will be so fully integrated into your body, that we won't even be able to see it.'

'Any questions?' breaks in El Presidenté mockingly.

'Sure Miss Mandela's got a question,' says the CIA man. ' "What's it going to *do* to me?" That's what you want to know isn't it?' He glances at the screen. 'Well, we're about to show you. OK Mr President. Whenever you're ready.'

El Presidenté picks up the remote control and presses the red button. Your whole body shudders. First there is just a kind of horrible involuntary twitching. Then, against your will, you rise out of the chair and towards the bowl of clotted cream. Your arms reach to pick up the bowl, your face drops into it your mouth opens, your tongue starts licking up the cream and you find yourself gulping it down. Then you start picking up handfuls of scone and stuffing them into your mouth. You realise the awful truth. The Fat Widow has taken control of your body.

El Presidenté is beside himself with joy, but still, between mouthfuls you bravely cry defiance.

'I'll tell the world what you've done!'

'Go ahead,' sneers the CIA man. 'No one will believe you. And try not to speak with your mouth full!' And with that you are pushed out into the street.

***

Your life is changed irrevocably. Every time El Presidenté presses the red button, you feel an incredibly powerful urge to eat, to stuff food into your mouth. You find that the autosacculina has been set so that with an immense effort you can resist. But once you are alone, the pressure of repeated pressings of the red button becomes unbearable and you chow down more food than ever. Sometimes El Presidenté gets bored and switches the control box to automatic. That is more predictable, but just as bad. Whenever you have eaten enough, the Fat Widow is triggered to urge you to eat more.

You become progressively more overweight. You try to maintain your public profile resisting the regime, but as your girth increases this becomes impossible. All your energy and time is devoted to fighting your personal battle against the Fat Widow inside you. In this private battle there is no longer room for a public role.

You go to doctors to try and get the Fat Widow removed. They take scans of your body but can find nothing. They think that you are deluded.

El Presidenté and the man from the CIA have defeated you far more surely than by bathing you in acid. Had you been murdered you might have become a martyr and symbol of resistance. But now, with your uncontrollable eating habits, you have merely become an overweight figure of fun.

***

Then, one day, you meet a doctor who listens unusually carefully to your story. He does not take a scan, instead he simply looks into your eyes for a long time.

'I believe you.' says the doctor. 'And I think I know the cure.'

'A cure?' You hardly dare to hope.

'Of all the strange things that they did,' says the doctor, 'the strangest of all is that they were completely open about it. They could easily have knocked you out, and you would have woken up with a scar and some story about appendicitis. But they did *not* do that. I think there was a reason; they wanted you to *know* what they were doing. Because once you know, you also know how powerful they are and how hopeless it is to fight them.'

'So I can do nothing?'

'No. There is something you can do. Ideally I would suggest that you try to forget all about what happened, but of course that's impossible, so instead try and remember it as a fantasy, something that you imagined, something that never really happened.'

'How?

'You believe in freedom?

'Of course.'

'Then I want you to free yourself. To do that you have believe that you are free. *I* know it really happened to you, but I want *you* to believe that, somehow, it didn't, that it was just some awful nightmare. And every time that filthy tyrant El Presidenté presses that red button, believe it again. Believe he's not there. Believe that you are free of him.'

'And then I can lose weight?'

'Yes. Try it and see.'

The doctor holds out a plate of cream buns. Somewhere El Presidenté presses the red button.

Your hand convulsively reaches out and clutches at a bun. 'It's just a fantasy!' prompts the doctor. 'Yes, It's a fantasy,' you manage to repeat. 'It's not real, there's no tyrant with a button forcing me to eat.' prompts the doctor. 'It's…not….real!' you gasp out. Slowly you release your grip and draw back your hand, empty. The buns lie uneaten on the table.

'Yes, it's working! I don't need to eat that bun!'

'It's not going to be easy,' said the doctor, 'but if you hold on to that belief, then you can do it.'

'Thank you doctor. Thank you so much!'

'You're very welcome. Goodbye, and good luck.'

'OK,' I said to the Guinea Pigs. 'You can all open your eyes. Now repeat after me:

'The story is a fantasy
There is no Fat Widow
No El Presidenté
Only me
And I'm free.
I can eat as much or as little food as I like.'

'I'm a bit confused,' said Angie. 'Are we meant to be imagining that the story is true or that it isn't true?'

'Sort of both,' I explained. 'You have to imagine that the story *is* true. Then that it *isn't* true. Even though you know in your heart that really it *is* true.'

'Though actually it isn't,' added Angie.

'The story isn't literally true, of course,' I said. 'But metaphorically it is true.'

'Why?'

It would not have been helpful at this point to give a wholly literal explanation for why the story was metaphorically true, so instead I turned to its philosophical context.

Imagination and Will

Let's take a step back and see what's going on with this story. Schopenhauer's Women's Diet exploits your ability to make physical changes to your body through your imagination and will. If you imagine something, and then *will* it hard enough, this can have a real impact on your physiology.

Take a tortoise. At some stage in the past tortoises did not have shells. What happened? Schopenhauer supplies the answer thus:

(a) they *imagined* shells and
(b) they *willed* shells, and so in the end
(c) they got shells.

If, therefore, you:

(a) *imagine* yourself losing weight and looking great and

(b) *will* yourself to lose weight and look great, then
(c) you will lose weight and look great.

Now, whatever we may think about tortoises, I think we can all agree that when it comes to dieting, Schopenhauer's argument is sound. If you have any doubts on this matter, consider something that is far harder to cope with than being overweight: cancer. There are some cancer patients who as well as following their doctor's advice have the indomitable attitude that they will fight the disease off and win. In fact they often die, but this by no means renders their attitude futile because they do tend to live longer than expected. Their determination, their will, has had a real physical impact in extending their life.

The comparison with people living with cancer tells us something else important. If an effort of will is to have an impact it cannot just be an ordinary effort. A casual vacillating effort of will is no good. It must be a forceful, concentrated, sustained and intense effort of will. This means that although Schopenhauer is right, his basic dieting advice on its own is useless because it is unrealistic; most people who are overweight are not going to make that concentrated rock-solid effort of will needed to lose weight. Their will to lose weight is about as firm as a hot air balloon tethered to the ground by a thin piece of rope. The balloon stays in places only until a small gust of wind snaps the rope and it takes off. The will to lose weight and look great stays in place only until the next bacon sandwich comes wafting by. Mmm delicious! Before you know it something snaps and you swallow the sandwich. Then you look around and wonder: 'Hey! Where's my will-balloon gone? Oh dear. Has it floated away *again*?'

This is where the realisation that the will is founded in the imagination is so important. If our will is weak, then perhaps by making more use of our imagination we can make it stronger. If we can tie the will to our imagination in lots of ways then we might stand a better chance of sticking to our diet and not having our will blown away every time we are tempted to eat more than we should.

By taking the story of the Fat Widow to heart and making it your own, you have already started to make new links connecting (a) your imagination to (b) your will to lose weight. Now you can (1) imagine losing weight and looking great but you can also imagine (2) that you have the Fat Widow inside you, then (3) you can imagine that really you don't. This gives your will-balloon, three 'ropes' connecting it to its foundations in the imagination, and this all helps to reinforce your will to reshape your body.

Imaginary Food

Now you are going to make your imagination stronger still, by making it active. You are not just going to sit and wait for tempting food to appear before imagining the Fat Widow. No, you are going to set out and actively seek food, engage with food, and in fact eat food, huge amounts of delicious fattening food, *in your imagination*. In other words you are going to pretend to eat food.

> Who can cloy the hungry edge of appetite
> By bare imagination of a feast?

asks Shakespeare's Richard II. The answer, of course, is that *you* can. You can snack on an imaginary banana, or spoil yourself with a slice of imaginary cake. You can even have a full-blown imaginary meal.

Like all aspects of imaginative dieting, while both men and women are welcome to give it a try it is much more likely to work if you are a woman. I have a friend who, as a teenager, would put tasty food into her mouth, masticate it, and then, at the point at which the food was ready to swallow, spit it out again. This she found surprisingly unsatisfactory. Now one might say that what she should have done was swallow the food and then make herself sick like Hobbes used to do. But in fact her mistake was to put the food in her mouth in the first place. If only she had trusted entirely to her ability to *imagine* eating, the result would have been very different! As Schopenhauer explains, women are just like children, in fact they 'remain children their whole life long.' This shows itself in all kinds of ways, but especially in 'taking appearance for reality.' In other words women, like children, have a very special and wonderful form of imagination. Any parent will know how a child finds it difficult to distinguish reality from their own fantasy. A child who reports a crocodile under the bed is not joking, they really believe it to be true. This marvellous imaginative gift is also held by women, and this is why a diet that blurs the distinction between fantasy and reality can be exceedingly effective for this sex.

Try eating a piece of imaginary food right now. You are going to have a snack, a very guilty snack: an entire 200 gram bar of fruit and nut chocolate.

> *The bar is in front of you, fully wrapped, in paper and in foil.* Tear *off the outer wrapping and* chuck *it on the floor. Who cares about litter! Now to the inner wrapping, the deep purple-blue foil. With the tip of your*

forefinger press down in the gap between the squares of chocolate, the foil bends and creases a little and then with a tiny gasp-like noise it splits, a barely perceptible tear. Now run your finger down between the squares pressing gently but firmly, until the tear becomes a thin slit that bifurcates the glittering foil giving you a glimpse the soft brown chocolate within. With the tips of your finger and thumb spread the foil back to reveal three or four full squares of rich creamy chocolate beneath. Now smell your fingers and delicately lick them to get the first faint chocolate taste. From one of the squares protrudes a hazelnut. Embedded in another you can make out the soft dark shape of a raison. Lift the chocolate bar to your lips and smell it deeply, just for a second, then take the first full bite. The chocolate breaks away and half fills your mouth. You chew as the chocolate begins to dissolve and flow down your throat, your tongue explores the firm edges of the hazelnut caught in the ridges of your molars, the raison yields its juice.

Now rip *back the foil to expose a large area of chocolate. Remember, it is yours, all yours. There is nothing to stop you scoffing the lot. This time take a really big bite, cram as much as you can into your mouth. Chocolate, hazelnuts and raisons in wild combination press against your inner cheeks and coat your tongue, mingle with your saliva and flow down your throat in great swallows. Take bites from the bar again and again, until the last small brown square disappears between your lips. Only the torn open foil remains. Screw this up and throw it to the ground. Now realise, with an intense rush of pleasure, that if you are not yet sated you can, if you like, eat another bar of chocolate, perhaps a white one or a dark, or even both at once in a kind of sandwich.*

That's the idea, now try to eat a piece of food using your own imagination.

***

Done eating? OK. A couple of things may have surprised you. First, you should have noticed your mouth salivating at the prospect of food. Second, you will find these meals to be surprisingly filling. Indeed you may well find that you are unable to finish the imaginary food you have started, or feel too full to eat more.

Eat whatever you like, but to heighten its effectiveness:

* Don't rush
* Imagine as much detail as possible
* Mimic the actions of eating

Once you have mastered eating imaginary food, Schopenhauer's women's diet is complete, and it is just a case of putting the pieces together. You can do this in your own way, but I suggest the following simple routine.

(1) When you wake up in the morning and again last thing at night, imagine a slim person, and say to yourself, with deep confidence, 'I am going to be like that.'

(2) Throughout the day whenever you feel like eating too much, remember that you are being forced to by El

Presidenté and his red button, then try and make yourself believe that this is just a fantasy.

(3) Eat as many imaginary snacks as you like!

Conversation with Derek

And that is where this chapter would have ended, if it were not for Derek. He hadn't participated in the session properly, just ogled the magazine, and when Angie and Jasmine went off together to buy some chocolate, he stayed behind.

'What did you make of the story Derek?' I asked.

'Yeah, that was great for the girls. But it wasn't my thing. I think I'm too much of a guy, you know what I mean?'

I recoiled slightly. Derek sounded friendly, almost as though he was reaching out to me after our recent spat. But if he thought that I was going to condone his way of life on the grounds that it was a 'guy thing' he could not be more mistaken.

'That El Presidenté story meant nothing to me,' Derek continued. 'I saw Jas and Angie writhing around as you were telling it, like they were really in to it, like they thought they were some kind of human rights hero. Well I ain't like that. I mean you've got to be pretty up yourself to imagine you're Nelson Mandela or whatever. Don't get me wrong. I believe in freedom. But the freedom in the story was do-gooder freedom, and what I mean by being free is not having no do-gooder telling me what to do. So basically the story was wasted on me. Like you said, the girls might imagine this stuff because girls are like kids. But men are Men.'

Throughout this little speech Derek's confidential and matey 'we're-all guys' tone had increasingly annoyed me. If he thought his unsavoury activities could be dignified by the name of freedom, it was time to put him straight by revealing something that I had thought best not to tell the others.

'Derek,' I replied, 'the story is what is called an "allegory" where the characters represent other things. And in that allegory, none of you were actually the hero or the heroine.' Here I chuckled. 'You weren't *really* imagining that you were noble and brave were you Derek?'

'You said we were. You *said* we was the hero.' (Derek had obviously been listening more than he let on.)

'Yes, Derek. I know I did. I was fibbing.'

'Oh "fibbing" are we Mr Philosopher? I though philosophy was the love of truth?'

'It is, yes. But in a dialectical philosophy truth can come out of error, and even lies.'

'OK. So if I'm not the hero in the story, who am I?'

'Do you remember that El Presidenté wiped his mouth clean before the Fat Widow was set loose?'

'Yes.'

'Well, actually he didn't; so when the autosacculina was released, El Presidenté mistakenly swallowed it himself.'

'I don't get it.'

'Don't you Derek? Can't you see what's staring you in the face? Of course you're not the hero Derek. *You're El Presidenté*. And the big red button you're pressing; *you're doing that to yourself*.'

I hadn't really intended to explain the real meaning of the story at this stage, but it had felt good to let Derek know a few home truths, and had he taken them in the right spirit of advice well meant then it might have done *him* the power of good too. But, of course, he didn't.

'You mean I'm the dictator?'

'Yes, the tyrant of your own body and you're torturing it, ruining it with your insatiable desire for food.'

'So underneath all the stuff about let's all be friendly and non-judgemental, that's what you think of us is it?'

'That's dialectics Derek.'

'Yeah, well I've had enough of it. I thought I'd give it one more try for Jasmine's sake, now me and Jas are going out, but you've fair turned me off.'

'I'm sorry that you think that way Derek,' I said, though actually I wasn't.

'And Derek,' I called out after him. 'The red button. It doesn't just apply to what you eat!'

The Women's Diet in a nutshell

* Eat Imaginary snacks.
* Whenever you reach for a *real* snack *it is not your fault*: El Presidenté is pressing his red button and *forcing you* to eat it. But if you pretend that El Presidenté does not exist you might be able to put the snack back.

Sources

C. Rossetti, *Goblin Market*
A. Schopenhauer, *Essay on Women*
A. Schopnehauer, *The World as Will and Representation*
A. Schopenhauer *The Will in Nature*

Chapter 8
Nietzsche's Uber Diet

which explains how to stop being űberweight.

Friedrich Nietzsche is the nastiest of all philosophers. He sneered at anyone he thought was unintelligent. He said that women should be treated like possessions and kept indoors. Worse than that, he wanted to breed a new caste of űbermensch, (supermen or 'overmen') to rule over the ordinary people of Europe. Nietzsche did not call ordinary people 'people,' instead he called them 'the herd' and said that the űbermensch should exploit and enslave them, use them as sadistic playthings, and kill them.

To try and justify this appalling idea, Nietzsche attacked Christianity, human rights and the nice philosophers Plato, Hobbes and Locke. Nietzsche despised Christianity because it said you should be kind to people, and especially the poor and the weak. And Christianity, Nietzsche said, was partly Plato's fault because he tried to get people to be good. Nietzsche also despised Locke's idea of human rights (which of course he didn't believe in), and he especially detested Hobbes's idea that we should all try and live peacefully together as equals.

There was another thing about Hobbes's philosophy that annoyed Nietzsche. Hobbes had said that you shouldn't laugh at other people, or rather, if you did, it was a sign of your own pettiness and inadequacy. Nietzsche, who *loved* to laugh at other people, seemed to take this as a personal insult. Of course it was not. How could it have been when Hobbes had died before Nietzsche was even born? But then Nietzsche was always seeing insults where none was intended, as poor Richard Wagner the opera composer found out. Wagner used to be a very good friend of Nietzsche, but grew increasingly anxious about his health. Now Wagner could have simply ignored the matter, but instead he acted like a true friend and did his best to help. He wrote a long letter to a famous doctor delicately explaining how Nietzsche masturbated *excessively*, and how this might be affecting him both physically and mentally, and could the doctor please do something about it? When Nietzsche found out about this letter, instead of being grateful to his kind-hearted friend he became churlishly angry about it, and took his revenge by spreading rumours that Wagner was Jewish. There is nothing wring with this of course—unless, like Wagner, you are a rabid anti-Semite.

At this point you may, understandably, be asking how this evil spiteful man could possibly help you to diet. It is a very fair question to pose, but look, before I start to answer it let us at least be *fair* about this. We should not be prejudiced against Nietzsche just because his philosophy is vile. He was, after all, very clever, and if we root around for long enough in the muck of his outpourings we may find a nugget of sound advice, the golden insight that we need to lose weight and look great. In fact you, the reader, are in the lucky position of not even needing to dirty your hands with Nietzsche because I have done it for you, and what is more, *I have found that lump of gold.*

You will want to know what this golden insight is, and I will tell you. But there is no point in telling you yet, because in order to *understand* Nietzsche's dieting advice, we must first make the acquaintance of a further nice philosopher, a genial Scotsman from the eighteenth century called David Hume, who Nietzsche found to be particularly stupid.

David Hume's Diet of Moderation

When it came to dieting Hume had a simple piece of advice:

Eat in moderation

Moderation means approaching meals with a sense of restraint, exercising self control and not eating too much. There is no need to cut rich foods out of your diet altogether, just limit how much you eat: have a little bit, and then stop. This advice is very old, Hobbes and Locke recommend it too, and moderation in eating is a part of the virtue that Plato calls 'temperance.' I have not mentioned it yet simply because (as all these philosophers also knew full well) while there is nothing actually wrong with this dieting advice, and while indeed it is obviously true, it is nonetheless *completely useless*. The only way in which a diet of moderation will work is if it is *combined* with some other idea or technique, hence Plato's getting back to nature, Hobbes's contract, and Locke's bucket.

Now poor Hume—perhaps he really was a bit dim—did not realise this. When he read these philosophers he thought that they meant that aiming to eat in moderation *on its own* was enough to keep to a diet and stay in shape. Then, to make matters worse, he caught completely the wrong end of the stick. Hume somehow got the idea that civilisation (which we know from Plato is making us more and more fat), is making us less and *less* fat, backing this absurd claim up with some irrelevant comment about how we no longer feast on raw horse like the uncivilised Tartars.* What a foolish mistake! The result was predictable, perhaps inevitable: Hume became hopelessly overweight.

* Hume failed to realise that if you spend your days racing bareback across the great Russian steppe and your evenings Cossack dancing, then you can basically eat as much as you like and still look great.

So fat did Hume become, in fact, that one day, when out walking near Edinburgh, he sank waist deep into a bog. Hume struggled gamely to escape but could not. So there he was. Stuck.

Sometime later, an old lady chanced to come by. Hume cried for help, and she pulled him out, but because he was an atheist she made him say the Lord's Prayer first.

Now while Nietzsche thought that Hume was right to be an atheist he also though that he was far too *nice* about it. Hume did not go around insulting believers and when it suited him he even pretended to pray, as he had done in the bog. Nietzsche, by contrast, was a *nasty* atheist. He went around saying 'God is dead,' and not just dead but *smelly*.

Criticising Hume for pretending to pray seems unfair. If he was going to get out of the mire, what else was he to do? But from a Nietzschean point of view, if Hume had not been so cowardly about his atheism he would not have got into this predicament in the first place. *For it was precisely because Hume was such a nice, cowardly atheist that he had grown so fat.*

As far as dieting was concerned, Hume would have been better off being a good Christian; he might have been deluding himself, but he would at least have believed that he had a duty to God to engage in self-denial and not to indulge his appetites whenever he felt like it. The great thing about Christianity is that it makes you feel *guilty* about this sort of thing. Whenever you sneak off for a furtive snack you know that someone is watching you disapprovingly: God. Once Hume stopped believing in God, he stopped feeling guilty. The thought of a sorrowful God tut tutting as you eat too much is, if you really believe it, a powerful incentive to stop. However, if like Hume you lack faith in God, then you cannot just replace Him with moderation. There is no point saying 'I don't believe in God, I believe in moderation instead.' Moderation does not promise Heaven and threaten Hell. Moderation has no awesome powers to perform miracles, no great cathedrals, no divinely inspired music. 'Moderation' is never going to save *anyone* from temptation.

The Philosophy of Excess

Nietzsche's solution to Hume's weight problem was that if you are going to be an atheist, then don't be content with half measures, don't just be a 'moderate' atheist—really go for it! Once there is no God, then there are no 'ten commandments' and in fact no morality at all. If, says Nietzsche, there is nothing to restrain you from doing what you want, then whatever you are doing, do it excessively, gratuitously, really *enjoy* it, *luxuriate* in it. It is no good having a philosophy of moderation; you must adopt a philosophy of *excess*.

Nietzsche's philosophy of excess may sound a little confusing. True it is quite different from Hume's diet of moderation in principle, but given that Hume was so fat, isn't it likely to be rather similar in practice? In other words, if you do things to excess, then won't you eat too much? It is a fair question, and the answer, as so often in philosophy, is going to be a little complicated.

Hume, let us remember, was a *nice* atheist. Now what does this mean? It means in effect that once Hume became an atheist he enjoyed doing the *little* things forbidden in Christianity, like overeating. However, Hume was by all accounts a pleasant fellow who was kind to his neighbours, which means that he did not do any of the *big* things that you ought not to do, like being cruel to people. Now according to Nietzsche, this was Hume's mistake, as to really be a consistent atheist, you must be nasty. Once you realise—really realise—that God is dead, then it is not just the little things that you can start doing without feeling guilty, *it's the big things too*. With God dead, all the things that you always wanted to do but didn't because they were 'wrong' or 'evil'—well now you can! And if you're willing to go for it and do those things, then you're an űbermensch or superman!

OK. Take a pencil, and tick the box that fits you best.

Are you:

(a) one of the űbermensch? ☐

or

(b) one of the herd? ☐

It's entirely your choice, but you do have to decide.

Chosen?

OK. If you've ticked the 'herd' box I want you to erase it and think again. I know that I have said that Nietzsche is not especially nice, but there is not need for you to be all prejudiced against his ideas. I might have been a bit unfair about the űbermensch too; they have a certain nobility about them, rather like big cats or, as Nietzsche put it, like 'blond beasts' tearing at the flesh of the herd. And perhaps even this is just a colourful metaphor, for he also described the űbermensch as artists, poets, musicians and mountain climbers; they are gifted, vigorous people. By contrast the herd are ordinary, all too ordinary. They are not at all like noble beasts of prey, but very like cows or sheep—peaceful but dim, exactly like a herd in fact. And did we not agree, at the very beginning of the book, that it was better to live for one day as a tiger than for a thousand years as a sheep?

Chosen again? Herd or űbermensch? If you are still one of the herd, then this diet is not for you. But if, and only if, you think you might an űbermensch, read on!

The Uberdiet in Four Easy Steps

Step 1: Admit it.
The first step in Nietzsche's diet is admitting to yourself that you are an űbermensch, You have now taken that very important step. Congratulations. What next?

Step 2: No guilt.
Did you feel a twinge of guilt when you admitted to yourself that you felt *better* than other people? *Well don't.* Nietzsche is very clear about this. If you *are* better than other people then there is absolutely no reason to feel guilty about it. You should feel good about your superiority. In fact, you should *revel* in it. It is only the herd that tries to make superior people like you feel guilty.

Step 3: Just do it!
Ask yourself this question: 'What *else* do the herd make me guilty about?' Whatever it is, then do it!

Step 4: Laugh at them.
Laugh at the herd for being like a herd.
And laugh at them *for being fat.*

At this point I can imagine you saying 'But I'm overweight myself.' But you won't be for long, not once you have freed yourself from herd-guilt.

Let's go back to Step Three. The fact is, the herd are *jealous* of you. They are envious of your potential, of your abilities. And they are *determined* to keep you in your place, to make sure that you are no better than them. That is why they try and make you feel guilty all the time; they *worm* their way into your brain so you are not even able admit to yourself how superior you are to those around you. No wonder you are frustrated. *No wonder that you eat too much.* That is exactly what they want. The herd want all űbermensch to be overweight. Only with overweight űbermensch do they feel safe. If you eat too much you will look just like them, the herd. If you eat too much you will even seem to *be* like them.

But you're *not* like them. And once you realise it and start to lose weight, then they are not safe.

The herd, like cows, are *naturally* fat. Their bovine stupidity lends itself to overeating and under exercising. They are happiest with other herd members waddling around the garden centre or shopping mall, or sat peacefully at home munching and staring at a screen, part of a great telly-watching herd. This makes them happy for they have no desire to be different, no ambition to be something more than they are.

Friedrich Nietzsche imagines life as a blond beast

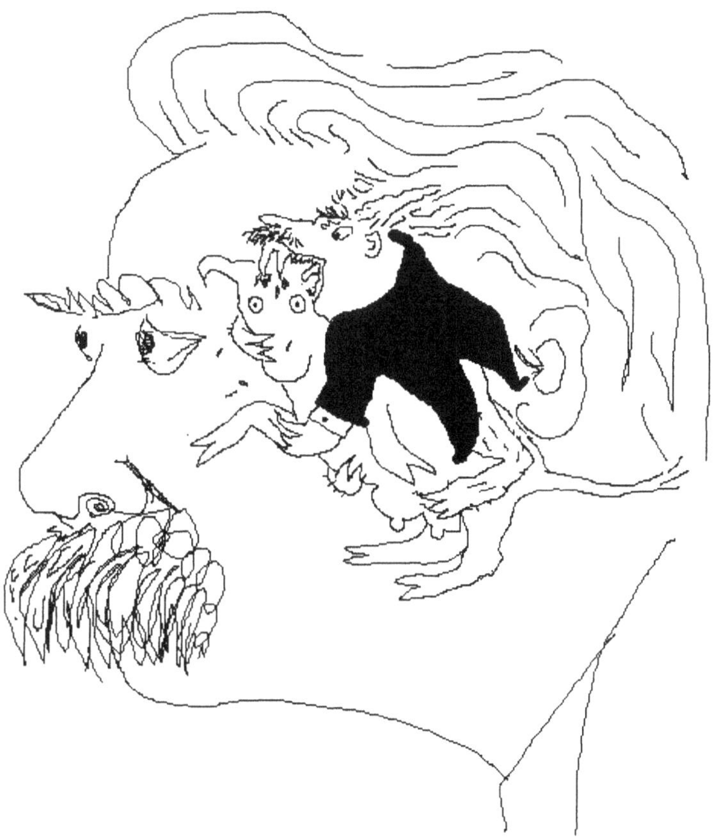

By contrast, űbermensch are *not* naturally overweight. No, the excess weight on an űbermensch are like chains that drag him—or her—down; the surplus flesh like a sponge soaking up the natural energy and dynamism of the űbermensch, the soft tissue like a cushion absorbing the űbermensch's hard edges and rendering him—or her—harmless.

Uberweight Ubermensch

If an űbermensch like you is overweight, what has gone wrong? The very word overweight gives us a clue. An űbermensch is an overman, but an overweight overman has turned everything that ought to put him or her 'over' other people into excess weight instead.

You, the űbermensch, have the drive to do some *thing*, a thing that is creative, exciting, dangerous. Whatever that *thing* is, the herd do not like it. It disturbs their comfort zone, their illusion that all 'humans' are equal. They have no creative potential, no willingness to take extraordinary risks, and they recoil instinctively from anyone who does as though they were a different species. So they do everything they can to block the űbermensch. They use guilt; they make up rules to stop whatever it is he or she wants to do; they bleat about human rights.

The űbermensch feels trapped and confused. There is no one they can turn to, no one who understands how they feel; they are alone in the herd. Constantly they are told that the very things that they aspire to are 'bad.' Yet they—you—have a powerful impulse inside them to do these 'bad' things. It demands to come out. It *must* come out. But the herd says that it *cannot* come out. The only way that the űbermensch can express this feeling is by doing something that satisfies the herd, because it is the kind of thing that the herd do themselves. But the herd do nothing that is creative, or exciting, or dangerous. And that is why, feeling lost and confused, the lonely űbermensch turns his or her colossal energies into overeating.

To follow the überdiet, therefore, you need to find your *thing* and do it to *excess*—just like Nietzsche did. Ignore the carping of well-meaning of friends trying to get you to stop, go ahead and get on with it. Live dangerously and creatively. Music, poetry, painting, mountain climbing and other things that require a vigorous imagination and a certain manual dexterity are all excellent examples. If you are not sure which of them is right for you, do them all: űbermensch have *lots* of abilities. As you develop your űbermensch excessiveness your weight will fall from you as naturally as autumn leaves dropping from a tree.

A Natural Diet

We need to pause and reflect here. You may have noticed that at the start of this chapter I said that Nietzsche's philosophy was about as nasty as one could get. But later on in the chapter I started encouraging you, the reader, to think of yourself as an űbermensch. This may seem a little irresponsible. Of course, it is fully in accord with philosophical dialectics to jump from one thing to its opposite and of course we are only talking about übermensch to help us go on a diet, not to breed a 'master race' to conquer the world and kill everyone. But isn't it a bit dangerous even to start thinking in this way?

Yes. I think that it is indeed dangerous. But I am not worried about getting you to think like that because I am guessing it is not a *new* thought. When it comes to feeling superior to other people, almost all of us think that way about ourselves *already*. I know I do. And I bet you do too.

The way in which most of us go round feeling superior was first noticed by Thomas Hobbes. Hobbes said that everyone went around imagining that they were better than almost everyone else. Hobbes explained that because *all* of us think like that, it really shows that we are all equal—equally conceited. He compared it to sharing out a cake and everyone happily imagining that *they* have the biggest piece, when really all the pieces were pretty much the same. Hobbes puts this in a rather funny way so that you end up laughing at yourself, but Nietzsche, who only liked to laugh at other people, must have been dreadfully annoyed by it.

Yet this appeal to people's smug sense of their own superiority is precisely why Nietzsche is such a popular philosopher. Instead of *challenging* people's conceit and prejudices, he *reinforces* them. Most people, in their hearts, spend their time feeling superior to other people and laughing inwardly at them, and Nietzsche justifies all this. 'My goodness!' they say to themselves, 'So *that's* why I have always felt I am more important than other people. It's because I'm an űbermensch!'

The great advantage of using Nietzsche, therefore, is that he provides a *natural* philosophical way to diet. There is not need to change the way you think or to conquer your worse feelings with better ones, none of that. You just affirm your perfectly natural, pre-existing feelings of complacent superiority about yourself and contempt for everyone else, and develop those feelings to help you lose weight.

As long as you restrict yourself to dieting there is no harm in this. The only unfortunate thing is that you are meant to laugh at other people for being fat and inferior. The problem with this (aside from its being cruel), is that it might spur *them* on to lose weight. And that is the *last* thing you want. But the solution here is to laugh at them in your head, and to laugh all the louder (though silently) because you are *tricking* them into becoming yet more overweight. It is easy enough to trick other people to gain weight. They are, after all, only stupid members of the herd. More particularly, they are like a herd of sheep, so we can trick them with a diet that we can call the 'sheep anti-diet.'

The Sheep Anti-Diet

At the start of Plato's *Republic* there is a character called Thrasymachus who tells a story about a shepherd and his sheep. The shepherd takes the flock to rich pasture where they eat lots of lush grass and grow fat. The sheep all think that the shepherd is being kind to him for finding them such nice food. But as a matter of fact the shepherd is fattening his sheep up so that he can take them to market. 'That,' says Thrasymachus, 'is how people behave. If they are stupid they are like the sheep, and if they are smart then they treat other people like sheep.' Plato said that this was a horrible idea and for thousands of years everyone agreed, until Nietzsche said that actually Thrasymacchus had been right all along and if you were smart you should indeed treat other people like sheep. How?—*by making them fat.*

OK. So we want to trick people into becoming more overweight: that's the philosophical principle that Nietzsche has picked up from Thrasymachus via Plato. But, how shall we actually go about doing this? What practical technique shall we use to get our 'sheep people' to overeat while *we* lose weight? This is not an easy question. After all, it is not as though you can force someone to eat more. So who might Nietzsche have turned to for the answer? Before I tell you, see if you can guess. Who was it that showed Nietzsche a practical way of tricking people?

Had a guess? OK. Now *I* want to guess two things:

(1) I bet you've guessed wrong.

(2) I bet that when I tell you the answer, you will kick yourself and say: 'Of course, it's obvious!'

Ready? Nietzsche got the practical idea of how to trick people from:

Drum Roll

Women

Clash of Cymbals!

That's right. The idea of tricking people into doing things they don't want to do comes from women. *They do it all the time.* They can trick people into just about anything, because that is what they are like: it's their nature.

I know. It is not a nice thing to say. And I personally don't believe it *for one minute.* But it is what *Nietzsche* said. He explained that because women were weak, they could not really force people (men especially) to do anything, so they tricked and manipulated them into doing things instead. How? By *seducing* them.

Now, of course, you do not have to go around *literally* seducing people in order to get them to overeat. But you can do similar things. Prepare some fattening food for them and look hurt when they do not take a second helping of it—while you eat a salad. Blow hot and cold—a classic seductive technique. Argue with them perhaps (cold) and then leave them chocolates in unexpended places (hot). I am not really sure what other advice to give, but I probably don't need to. Because the really exciting thing is that if Nietzsche is right, all you have to do as a woman is to *be yourself.*[*] As a woman you will instinctively *know* what to do. You don't actually need me to tell you anything, you will work out a way. You are already an accomplished seductress! And this makes the űberdiet even more natural for you.

From Guinea Pigs to Ubermensch

Streaks of dawn radiated from a smudge on the horizon like the whiskers of a cat that had inadvertently puts its nose into a pot of pink paint while searching for salmon. I loved this time of day, the cool air, the grass and ferns wet with dew. And the two remaining Guinea Pigs, Angie and Jasmine, what would they think of it? Nietzsche was very keen on űbermensch singing from mountain tops, so in pursuit of the űberdiet we were going to climb a mountain and improvise poems when we reached the summit. But, as of yet, I was still on my own down in the car park. I had arrived a little early, when would they come?

Beep! –It was a text message from Jasmine.

cant cum cat sick j ☹

My heart leapt though I hardly knew why. It was something I had barely admitted to myself. Angie, just Angie, and this beautiful dawn!

no probs thanx for letting me no p ☺

[*] If you are a man, hard luck.

Beep! –Now one from Angie. Great! Probably to say she was on her way.

cant cum js cat sick a ☹

wot do u mean u cant cum surely she cn look after her own bldy cat p ☹

she nds emotional spprt

well wot about drk

out late last nite and still in bd

alright well after drk wakes up then cud u cum

ok

☺

Eventually, around lunchtime, Angie did indeed turn up. Together we climbed the mountain. Together we improvised poems and shouted them into the wind. And on the way down, I let my tongue run wild with more poetry. Angie was a goddess, divinely beautiful, supremely intelligent, creative, life affirming. It was as if searching amongst the clay of humanity, I had found a precious stone. I did not want to lose this jewel from my grasp, I wanted to polish it clean, cherish it, gaze into it.

Angie received this with guarded interest. She resisted my suggestion that we do some more stomach rubbing, allowing me only to hold hands. She said would think about it.

And in the meantime, she said, I ought to make amends to Derek and Stuart. Both of them, she told me, were suffering from low self-esteem. That was partly the result of being overweight, yes. But it was partly my fault too. Stuart had been trying very hard to diet to gain Wendy's approval. But every time he took my advice, things kept going wrong. And Derek had come away from the Women's Diet feeling mortally offended.

I am, I hope, big enough to take criticism. So that very night I phoned Derek and I phoned Stuart. I apologised whole-heartedly, and I invited them to a man's meeting, 'no girls allowed,' where I would tell them things about dieting that would help them lose weight, and would also make them feel much better about themselves.

My idea was simple, I would introduce them to the űberdiet, and explain that *they* were űbermensch. To make this rather unlikely claim more convincing, I would take a leaf out of Schopenhauer's women's diet and use my imagination. I would talk to Stuart and to Derek, but in my mind, I would *imagine* I was talking to Angie.

This worked remarkably well, though I should add that I can take no credit for persuading Stuart and Derek to embrace their instinctive feeling that that they were superior to everyone else; the praise belongs entirely to Hobbes for his extraordinary psychological intuition into how people think. I was also reminded of Descartes and the relationship between the mind and the body, for if you can believe something in your mind, then that is half the battle. By the end of the session there was a new can-do confidence about them, an impression of irrepressible self-esteem, and a lack of esteem for others.

Derek admitted he had been shaken when I had told him that, philosophically speaking, he was no better than the tyrant El Presidenté, and was relieved when I informed him that in fact he was an űbermensch.

'So all that stuff you were saying to me was kind of a test?'

'Exactly.'

'Sort of like at the start? I mean when Knud pretended to storm out to make it seem like we wouldn't be on TV anymore, when really we still are.'

'Yes. Something like that, yes.'

'You know Pete, you almost fooled me. I was about ready to settle down and become part of the herd!'

'Don't do that Derek. The way you've lived your life has been an instinctive embodiment of the values of the űbermensch. Now you *know* that you're an űbermensch you can now really start to enjoy it. Guilt free. No holds barred. Make the most of that strong will you've got. And once you stop feeling guilty about it, I guarantee you'll lose weight.'

'Crikey, Pete, perhaps you're right, I mean that's what half of me's been saying to myself anyway.'

'That's the űbermensch inside you Derek. Listen to that voice and you can't go wrong.'

'So, when I've been feeling guilty, thinking I should behave properly, like what my grandma would have wanted me to, I mean, I shouldn't…?'

What you should or should not do is down to you. But is the strait-laced morality of your grandmother really appropriate for free spirits like you? Don't you feel suffocated by all that kind of stuff? Ubermench aren't tied down by petty moral codes. Set sail for uncharted waters, break your chains.

Live how *you* want to live. Enjoy everything. No restraint, no small-minded curtain twitching. Go for it.'

'You really think I'm an űbermensch?'

'It's obvious. Just look at you—how handsome you are.'

'Handsome?'

'*Inner* handsomeness Derek. You're incredibly charismatic, incredibly alive, it shines out of you like a light. Powerful too.'

'Do you think so?'

'Gosh yes. Remember how you threatened to thump that guy Steve? When he was going to throw a cream pie in your face? I mean one *look* from you, and he backed right off.'

'Yeah, I suppose.' Derek chuckled at the memory

'Use that power! That charisma. Live life to the max.'

Derek stared into the middle distance.

'Yeah,' he said thoughtfully.

'Atta Boy!' I said encouragingly, and thumped him on the shoulder in a one-űbermencsh-to-another kind of way. 'And remember this.' I turned to the whiteboard and wrote in large capital letters:

GOD IS DEAD

So much for Derek. Next I turned to Stuart, who had been listening to all this agog.

'You're an űbermensch too Stuart,' I said decisively and confidently.

Stuart looked relived.

'Am I really? I thought I might be one of the herd.'

'No way Stu. Ubermensch through and through. I can tell. Underneath the surplus flesh you have the body of a Greek God. Don't let them seduce you into thinking you're part of that herd. You're a beast of prey!'

'Seduce me?'

'Yes, seduce you. You're a dangerous man of action and they're using food to tame you…'

As I explained the Nietzscehan concept of 'seduction' to Stuart, his mouth started to hang open, and his eyes grew rounder and rounder. Suddenly he interrupted me.

'Oh My God!'

'Yes?'

'It's Wendy. *Wendy's* been seducing me!'

'Wendy?'

'Yes! She's *always* buying me things to eat. She puts them in the fridge where she *knows* I'm going to find them.'

'Why would Wendy…?'

'It's obvious isn't it? She wants to stop me being an űberman, like what I naturally am. And she doesn't like me exercising. She wouldn't let me buy a jet ski the other day.'

Stuart, as usual, had not grasped things as fully as he might have done. But I let it pass. He had got the basic idea and the next I heard he was indeed jet skiing—close to the shore on a beach popular with small children.

Later, the Vicar phoned to complain again: Why had 'God is dead' been written in large capital letters on the whiteboard in the church hall? The cubs, who had come in afterwards, were asking questions about it.

'And don't go pretending it is another "accident" either,' he added petulantly.

I told the Vicar that accident or no I was *glad* that the cubs had seen it as I believed it was good for young people to question the things they were taught, especially if it happened to be outdated superstitious rubbish. We had another argument, which ended, as it always did, with the Vicar saying said that we could never use the church hall again. This time, however, I let him have his way. Our meetings had reached a natural end point anyway. My gamble in introducing the Guinea Pigs to the Four Germans had paid off, and I had more than enough material for the book I wanted to write. Overall, I felt that I had finally achieved success. Wendy was now slim. I had restored the self-esteem of the male GPs. And in Angie I hoped I had found a new relationship.

Everything had gone so well that I decided that I may as well try Jasmine on the űberdiet too. But she was the only one I had trouble with. Jasmine was almost as dim as Stuart, which in one way made my task harder, because it made the suggestion that she was really an űbermensch particularly preposterous. In another way, however, it ought to have made things easier, because she should have been easier to persuade that it was true. However, try as I might, Jasmine refused to admit that she was superior to other people. No matter what argument I used and what superlatives I applied to her (imagining her to be Angie), she would just shake her head and say 'No, I don't think that's right.' She also seemed unaccountably upset about something. In the end, I gave up and put her back on the laughter diet to cheer her up.

The Uberdiet in a Nutshell

1. Do not feel guilty about thinking that you are superior to everyone else—you are! Act accordingly.
2. Trick other people into eating too much.

Sources

D. Hume, *A Treatise of Human Nature*
D. Hume, 'Of Refinement in the Arts'
F. Nietzsche, *The Gay Science*
F. Nietzsche, *Beyond Good and Evil*
F. Nietzsche, *The Will to Power*
Plato, *Republic*

Part 3
Crime and Punishment

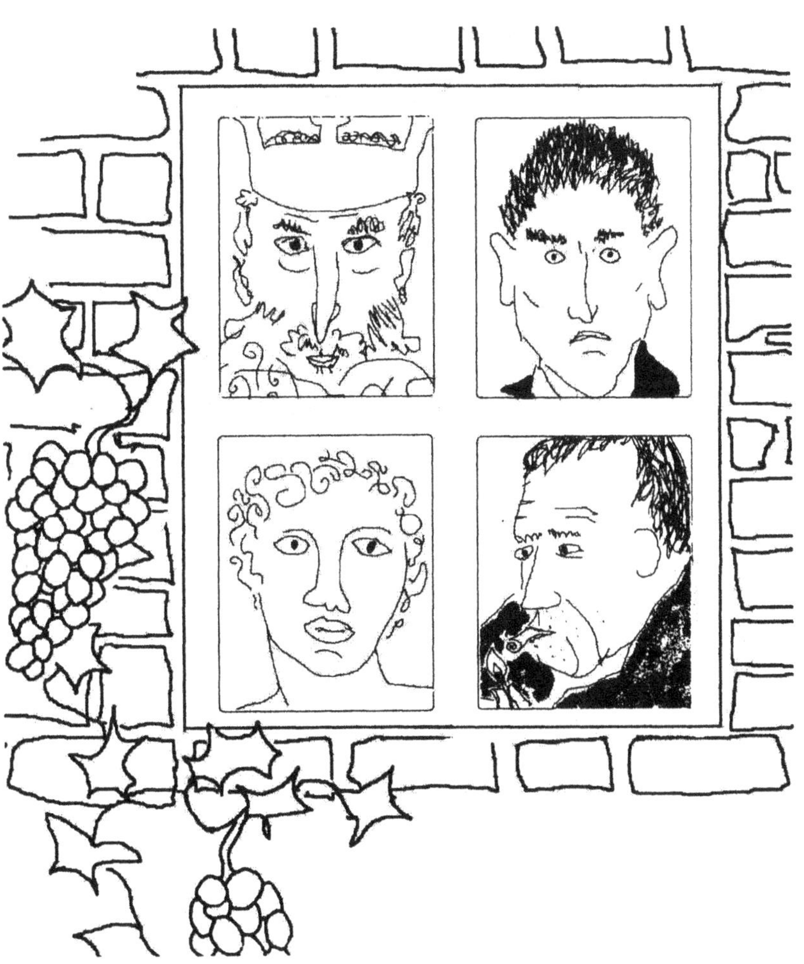

Chapter 9
The Trial

which explains why being overweight is your own fault.

It is said that Mozart composed his Jupiter Symphony in sixteen days. This was a record that I was determined to beat for the book I was about to write, at least in its first draft. I explained to Angie how sometimes I needed to be totally at peace and alone, and that this was one of these times (thesis). She said fine. She was busy floor sanding with Jasmine and didn't want to see me either (antithesis). There was a hurt edge to her voice which made me yearn for our synthesis. But what I said was true: I needed to concentrate, and my creative juices could not be channelled off elsewhere. Chopin had the same kind of problem fending off George Sand, and I expect Hobbes did with Mary Dell.

I prefer to write by hand, and so for the first draft of my book I took myself off to the woods with pen and paper. I found a comfortable spot, started to write and *The Philosophy of Dieting* rapidly began to take shape.

The glade where I wrote each day was close to a track frequented by Wendy. I would often hear her singing and then, as I sat motionless, see her padding past me in her bare feet. Wendy now had a fetching wood-fairy figure—the diet of pigs had reached into her very soul and transformed her. But despite my success in finding the right diet for Wendy, a certain coolness seemed to have developed between us, so I refrained from saying anything to her.

One day as Wendy walked past she noticed me quietly sitting there. Her face flushed and she backed away like a startled deer. I thought that I had seen the last of her, but two days later, as I was putting the final touches to the manuscript, she came back. She smiled at me shyly, rather like a deer again.

'Hello Peter.'

'Hello Wendy! My, look at that svelte body! You look fantastic! How's Stuart?'

'Oh, his tapeworms are nearly all gone now.'

'Super!'

'Yes. We got quite fond of them in the end, almost like pets.'

'Well, I suppose people keep snakes.'

'Exactly.'

'I had a hamster once.'

'Did you Pete? How very sweet.'

'So he's feeling fit and well again?'

Yes, kind of, at least he's stopped jet skiing after the accident.'

An accident? I'm sorry to hear that.'

'Luckily he didn't hit anyone, just landed on his nose.'

'That's a relief.'

'Yes, it makes him look quite handsome, a bit like Al Pacino.'

'Well, that's sort of turned out quite well then too.'

'Yes. Anyway Pete, I hoped I'd find you here. We're all having a barbecue and we'd really like you to come. Bring your notes along: we'd love a "sneak-preview".'

As I say the draft was almost done and it seemed churlish to disagree, so I accepted the invitation and went straight back with Wendy to her home, which bordered on the woods. Wendy took my manuscript and poured me a drink and I wandered out into the garden. In the middle of the lawn a table had been laid out with familiar looking cakes and buns and near the end of the garden was a blazing fire. Around the fire stood the Vicar's wife, Stuart, Jasmine and Angie. Angie! Outwardly calm, my suppressed emotions surged through me like an earthquake.

The GPs waved brightly and beckoned me over, though as I approached I saw that the girls were smiling in a slightly strange way. Stuart, who looked anxious, started shifting from one foot to the other and biting his finger nails.

I had assumed that it was woodfire going, but as I soon saw that it was not. The Guinea Pigs were not burning wood, they were burning books. Diet books. A considerable number were already alight, and others were being tossed into the blaze.

'What's up GPs?' I asked curiously.

'We've all got loads of them cluttering up our shelves, and we've decided we don't need them anymore because, basically, they're all crap,' explained Angie as she threw a best selling book that promised to make you thin into the flames.

I laughed genially, while inside a thrill ran though my body like an aftershock at the sound of Angie's voice.

'Well, maybe that's a little harsh Angie' I said, 'But I see what you mean. And you're essentially right of course: they're all useless, and once *my* book is published then....'

The words died on my lips. Wendy had followed me into the garden and now stood on the far side of the fire. She was holding my manuscript, and she was looking between it and the flames in a meaning kind of way. Then Wendy looked through the smoke at me and smiled. Her smile did not at all remind me of a shy deer, she looked more like a crocodile. I tried to move round the fire towards her, but Angie was blocking me on one side, and Jasmine was on the other. The

Vicar's wife was looking on quizzically, while Stuart was hopping about in the background nervously nibbling the rim of a custard pie.

'Wendy?'

Wendy waved the manuscript threateningly.

'Stay there Peter! Or it all goes in at once.'

'Be careful Wendy, it might catch light and I've spent weeks working on it…'

'Silence in court!' exclaimed Wendy

'Court? Wendy what are you doing? Guinea Pigs, what's going on?'

I turned to the others. Stuart had buried his face in his pie and the faces of Angie and Jasmine were hard and unsympathetic. They said nothing, but Wendy cleared her throat and read the title page of my manuscript in a 'plummy' tone of voice that I think was meant as an imitation of my own:

' "The Philosophy of Dieting by Peter Hayes, PhD".' Then she peeled the page off and tossed it into the fire.

'Wendy!'

' "Acknowledgements",' read Wendy, now in a sarcastic tone of voice.

' "It is a bit funny writing these acknowledgements" ' she read, ' "because it is actually these guys who should be acknowledging me. Still, I suppose I ought to thank the five Guinea Pigs who have tested the diets I taught them. They have proved that you don't need to be smart to benefit from philosophical dieting. In fact, providing you can grasp a few simple philosophical principles, you can actually be quite dim, and still lose weight and look great".'

'It's only a draft, I might rewrite that bit.'

Wendy ignored me and kept on reading.

‘ “So thank you Angie, Wendy, Stuart, Jasmine and Derek. You guys are an inspiration to ordinary people everywhere!” ’

Wendy tossed this page onto the fire too. Then she asked:

‘Why shouldn’t I burn the rest of it?’

I felt like I had slipped into a nightmare or horror film and it took all my courage not to cry out or to run.

‘Burn it?’

‘Yes. It’s all rubbish isn’t it?’

It was the age old reaction of the mob against philosophy. I remembered Hobbes and how must have felt when the bishops were burning *his* books, and I remembered the bravery of Socrates whose philosophy had cost him his life. In a small way I realised that I was now becoming a part of that noble tradition of philosophers who defied violent superstition with sober rationality, and this gave me strength. I took a deep breath. I was determined to stay calm. When I spoke it was in my normal voice, or rather it was in my ‘foreigner voice,’ by which I mean the slow, distinct and encouraging kind of voice that I use when conversing with people who are learning to speak English, and who have not yet got very far.

‘No. It is not rubbish. But even if it was, you should not burn it, because I am a *guest* at your barbecue?’

‘You’re not our guest,’ spat Wendy.

‘More like a defence lawyer,’ explained Angie. ‘We’ve got your book prisoner, and we’re putting it on trial.’

‘On trial? Why?’

‘I ask the questions!’ cut in Wendy sharply, ‘and I’ll ask you again. What makes your book any better than all this other rubbish?’

'The manuscript, my book, and these other books are two completely different things Wendy,' I replied. I gestured to the pile of yet unburnt books by the fire. 'Those books feed people's illusions, my book will teach people to understand reality. It is not just about dieting; it is a book that will save democracy from sinking under its own weight. Look, I know that these diets have been hard on you, all of you, because you are just ordinary people who are not used to philosophising. But if you burn my manuscript, you are not just burning bits of paper, you are rejecting everything you have learned, everything you have gained.'—Wendy snorted. 'You may not always have understood the deeper philosophical implications of the diets we have been trying,' I continued, 'but you ought to be able to see the benefit if explaining them to others. This is a book to *help* people. Like it has helped you.'

'Helped us!' exploded Wendy.

'Yes Wendy, helped you: you have lost weight haven't you? Well that is all due to me.'

'And what about Stuart?' Wendy was shouting with anger, 'He's been whipped, arrested for loitering; hospitalised! And now,' Wendy said, her voice rising to a crescendo of fury, 'you've been trying to destroy our marriage by telling him that I'm "seducing" him into being fat! Is *that* all due to you too?'

'No Wendy,' I said, slowly and calmly. 'That is *not* due to me. All of that is *Stuart's* fault.'

Stuart made a sort of squeaking noise and twiddled the soft central core of his uneaten custard pie. Wendy lifted the manuscript above her head hurl it on to the fire. I closed my eyes.

'Wait!' cried Angie.

'Wait up Wendy, this is meant to be a fair trial; let him explain why he thinks it's Stuart's fault. If he doesn't convince us, then you can chuck it in.'

'Thank you Angie,' I said. 'I will explain. But it involves another diet. Do you mind if I sit down?'

Franz Kafka

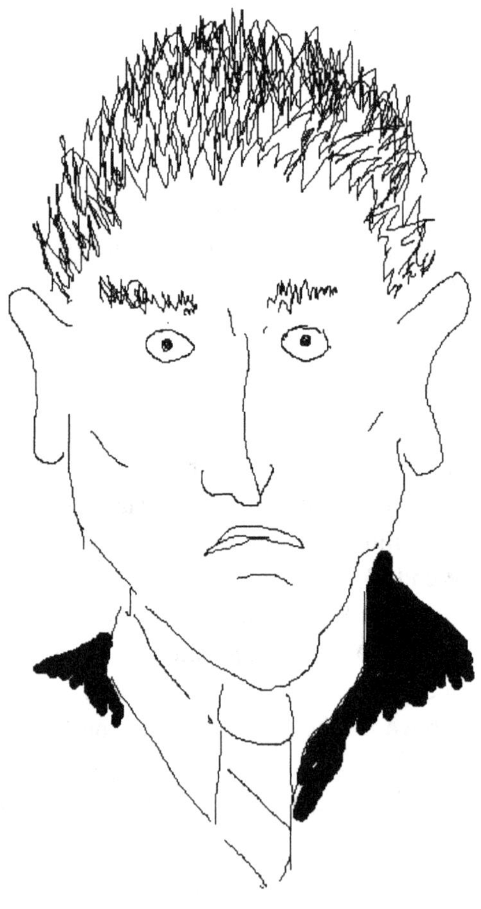

Kafka's Trial Diet

'I did not think that I would have to tell you this diet, I explained to the four Guinea Pigs and Vicar's wife, 'or rather, I did not want to tell you directly; I thought it was better to hide it in the laughter diet.'

'What do you mean hide it?' asked Angie suspiciously.

'It's dialectics.' I said, then seeing the blank looks I added, 'You have to move towards the truth slowly, sometimes. If it all comes out too quickly, it can be painful. There is a wonderful scene in *David Copperfield** where a teacher tells a child that his mother is dead, but he does it gradually, so as not to upset him. I was doing something a bit like that.'

'Treating us like kids now!'

'Exactly! Yes. You've got the idea.'

But my explanation of dialectics only angered the girl Guinea Pigs more, and accusations burst forth first from Wendy and then Angie in a kind of duet.

'We're not children, we're adults!'

'Wasted our time for months.'

'Always lying!'

'Not telling us things properly.'

No wonder your rotten diets don't work!'

'No wonder I'm still fat!'

This last comment was relative; when I arrived in the garden I had been gratified to see that Angie and Jasmine both appeared slightly slimmer than when I had last seen them. But I conceded the point. 'Alright,' I said, 'I understand that you believe that it is my fault that—Wendy aside—all of you

---

* By Charles Dickens.

continue to be overweight? Well, maybe it is. Certainly, I cannot deny that I have been toning the philosophers down for you, making them sound softer and nicer than they really are, and I suppose that that is a bit like treating you as children. So now I am going to do what I can to make amends. I am going to tell you the plain truth.'

'Maybe you should have done that earlier,' said Angie.

'Maybe I should, but better late than never.'

'That won't get you off the hook,' said Wendy.

'Actually,' I replied, 'it has not been *me* that has been on trial for the last few months. The philosophy of dieting has been an experiment, a process a bit like a medical trial, with the diets like doses of different drugs. You Guinea Pigs have been the volunteers to test whether or not they work, and whether they have any unpleasant side effects. But have you ever asked yourselves why you entered the trial in the first place? I will tell you. You entered it because you thought it *was* going to be a bit like that pile of books that you are burning. You hoped that you would find some dieting philosophy that would prove that *being overweight is not your fault*. But the problem is that the philosophers tell you the opposite. Being overweight *is* your fault. You have eaten too much and exercised too little. Often you have done this in secret, as if by hiding it from other people you can hide the truth from yourself. And you have chosen to do that. You have chosen to be fat. That is the 'adult' truth, the unpleasant truth, the philosophical truth. And *that* truth,' I concluded, 'is why you don't like philosophical dieting and want to burn my book.'

There was a stunned silence at this little speech. It had a particular effect upon Stuart, I could tell, because he had forgotten completely to eat the middle bit of his pie, even thought it was the best part.

I let the silence hang in the air for a second or so and then went on.

'I want to tell you a story. A true one. In Kierling in Austria in 1924 Franz Kafka lay in a hospital bed. He was still quite young, but he was dying of tuberculosis. In his final hours Kafka called in his best friend, Max Brod, and told him the location of a manuscript he had been working on. He asked him to guard it carefully and, if possible, to get it published.[*] That manuscript went on to become the greatest philosophical novel of the twentieth century: *The Trial.*

'What is the novel about? It *appears* to be about an innocent man called Joseph K caught up in an endless secret trial in some kind of totalitarian regime—this is how the book is usually read today. But it is a misreading. In fact Joseph K is guilty. Guilty of what? Guilty of *participating* in the trial. Guilty of keeping it a *secret*. Guilty because he does not admit that the trial is his *own fault*. Guilty because he *chooses* to be guilty.'

'Now you asked me why I said that Stuart, and not I, was guilty. In a sense I have been Stuart's accuser, I could even be said to have been persecuting him like Joseph K was apparently persecuted. But I have never *forced* Stuart to do anything. Stuart did not have to frequent public toilets, eat tapeworms, and blame his wife for plotting to make him fat, he *chose* to do it for himself.'

Stuart listened intently, his brow furrowed, his uneaten pie sagging from his fingers.

---

[*] I should mention to the reader that this is not *exactly* true; Kafka actually gave instructions to Brod to burn all his manuscripts.

'There's a scene in *The Trial* when a man wants to get through a doorway. The door is open, but a gatekeeper is there and he tells the man that he cannot pass. But this is not true. Really the man can pass by easily, all he has to do is one simple thing: ignore the gatekeeper. But he never does, and in the end he dies, still on the wrong side of the door.

'When you embark on a diet you want to get though that door, and I want to help you through it. I want you to take control of your life, and when someone orders you to do something unreasonable, whether that person is me, or your own internal voice demanding too much food, I want you to have the courage to break free, say no; to step through that door.

'But especially I want Stuart to take that step.'

Stuart looked offended in a 'why-pick-on-me?' way.

'Because Stuart, you must admit, is impressionable,' I continued. 'He does what Wendy tells him; he does what I tell him. He believes things. He lacks independence. He needs to find that independence if he is to lose weight. And so, from early on in our meetings, I have become Stuart's gatekeeper.

'I have stood by the gate that Stuart needs to pass, openly telling him one thing, while silently willing him to defy me. I have told him or hinted to him to act in ways that are absurd. But never once has he stepped through the door and become his own person. Never has he yet gained the freedom of mind to take his own course.

'So it is true, in a sense, that I did encourage him to do all those things: the tapeworm, the whipping, the toilet debacle, blaming Wendy for his snacking habits. I persuaded him to leave Wendy in San Francisco too. But all the time, I was willing him to say no, to revolt, to stop being such a wimp!'

Stuart was staring at me open mouthed, his face working with some deep seated emotion. Then in a dramatic forceful gesture, he rushed over to me and squashed the remains of the custard pie into my face.

'Congratulations Stuart,' I said. 'You have finally stepped through the door.'

The Trial Diet in a Nutshell.

* You have chosen to be fat.
* Make another choice: Eat less and exercise more.
* Don't eat in secret.

Source

Franz Kafka, *The Trial*

Chapter 10
Camus' Rebel Diet

which explains why you should keep trying to diet even when it is pointless.

There was a moment of stunned silence. Then Jasmine and Angie broke out into a spontaneous round of applause. The Vicar's wife slapped Stuart on the back, and Wendy hugged him. I cleaned my face and then gently asked if I might now have my manuscript back. Wendy hesitated for a moment, and looked to Stuart. He nodded his assent, and she started towards me with it.

Jasmine intercepted her. 'I'll take this please.' She held the manuscript tightly to her bosom, her long nails gleaming as they bit into the paper.

This looked worrying, but surely Jasmine had nothing to complain about, or at least not very much.

'Those are beautiful nails Jasmine,' I lied cautiously, trying to feel my way towards what her problem might be.

'Thank you' said Jasmine. 'Do you know who I met this morning when I was having them done?'

'No. Who?'

'Sharon' she said.

'*Who*?'

'Sharon.'

'I don't think I know anyone called "Sharon".'

'Yes you do. Don't you remember? She was in the A Team. Used to work in a pub.'

Then it came back to me. Of course, Sharon, the blunt yet emotional working class lass, one of the ones Knudson wanted to film dieting, despite the fact that she already had a great body, probably because she smoked.[*]

I could see what was coming, and broke in quickly to pre-empt it.

'Guinea Pigs, guys, listen. I have a confession to make. That stuff about the documentary, about how the A team were on some island paradise. I made it all up. I wasn't lying. It was dialectics again.'

The Guinea Pigs were staring at me mystified.

'But didn't you…? Angie began.

I interrupted again.

'No. Look, I'm sorry if you're disappointed. I always meant to tell you. I was just waiting for the right time: the time when you were ready to pursue philosophy for its own sake. Well, I think that time is now. So I'm glad to get things straightened out. After I chose you to do the diet and the A team left, they all just went home. There's no documentary, No TV, no Knud.'

'But there *is* a documentary!' Jasmine exclaimed.

'What?'

'The thing is, we're not in it,' added Stuart.

It was my turn to look mystified.

'A "documentary?" What do you mean?'

'Didn't you know? It started on telly last night. Look.'

Jasmine pressed a button on her smart phone, and passed it to me, and with a sickening shock, I watched the show unfold.

---

[*] Do not smoke as a method of dieting.

TRANSCRIPT 3

(Jazzy saxophone music. Pictures of famous philosophers interspersed with clips of the A Team larking about. ROSEMARY and SHARON dance barefoot; STEVE tries to climb a coconut tree; TANSU holds a live lobster dangerously close to FOGGY's bottom.)

TITLE: The Philosophy of Dieting
SUBTITLE: With Knud Knudson

EXTERIOR. Beach. Blue sky. Breeze.

KNUDSON: (walking along the beach) We all need to diet. But what is the philosophy of dieting? Well, we are going to find out.

(More Jazzy music and A Team frolics)

KNUDSON: Philosophy has a reputation for being dull, abstract and boring: a dry academic subject taught by fat professors in woolly sweaters.

(A picture of a professor is briefly flashed onto the screen. His face is blacked out, but I am fairly certain he is me. Certainly I have a sweater of that pattern.)

KNUDSON: But philosophy doesn't have to be like that. Philosophy started in Ancient Greece and the Greeks certainly were not fat. Maybe we can learn something from them.

(Shot of a marble statue of a nude APHRODITE. The camera zooms in on her face. Then slowly and lasciviously it moves down and around her body.)

KNUDSON: (voiceover) The most famous Greek philosopher was Aristotle, and he lived off seaweed. So for our first lesson in the philosophy of dieting we are collecting seaweed too.

(APHRODITE fades into TANSU who is kneeling over a large rockpool and reaching down into it. STEVE looks on. SHARON smokes on a nearby rock. In the background FOGGY is snorkelling.)

FOGGY: (rising from the sea with a scalp of kelp clutched in his fist) Yo guys! Breakfast!

(ROSEMARY supervises FOGGY as he gambols about building a fire on the beach to cook the seaweed.)

KNUDSON: (standing by the fire chewing seaweed) Seaweed may be healthy but it can also be dangerous. In fact, more people die from seaweed than from shark bites. One day, on a beach very like this one, Aristotle was out collecting seaweed when he slipped over and...

TANSU: (falls into the rockpool) SCREAMS.

(ROSEMARY and FOGGY race urgently down the beach. STEVE hops about on the rocks not sure what to do. SHARON tosses her cigarette onto the sand and slips languidly out of her t-shirt.)

I switched off. I could not bear it any longer. I was stunned by the duplicity of someone I had thought of as a friend. I returned Jasmine's smartphone, pulled out my own rather more primitive mobile and dialled furiously.

'Hello Peter. Did you like the show?'

'Knudson you lying shit! You've stolen my idea!'

'Not "lying" Peter. Dialectics.'

Knudson did not laugh very often, but when he did it was a noisy and prolonged affair. Now, out of the phone, came the reverberations of deep hearty laughter. He sounded like Jove must have done after he had castrated Saturn.

I switched the phone off and stared deeply into the fire.

'What can I say GPs? Knudson's betrayed me. And he's got it all wrong; Aristotle didn't eat seaweed; he was studying it.'

'*You* feel betrayed?' said Jasmine. So do we. *We* went on all these diets. Had a rotten time. And then *they* turn into celebrities. Sharon's already been getting all kinds of offers: adverts, nightclubs, tobacco companies. It's just not fair.'

'I'm sorry Jasmine.'

'All those stupid things you suggested. And it wasn't just Stuart who had to go to hospital. I had to go to hospital too when you said if I made myself sick I'd look like Princess Diana. And for what? It all—well it all just seems so pointless. Why put us through all of that for nothing?'

'Not for nothing. I mean it's true you're not on TV, but you have made friends; you've made rather *good* friends with Derek,' I insinuated. 'Where is he anyway?'

The fire flared a vivid swollen red and a great cloud of black smoke billowed out and surrounded us, stinging our eyes and making us cough and splutter.

Jasmine started to cry.

'Oh Peter!' exploded Angie throwing her arms protectively around her friend. 'Throw it in the fire Jasmine. The Bastard! "Where's Derek" indeed! You must know where he is. And it's all your fault. Go on Jasmine, rip it up, chuck it in!'

But Jasmine was not listening. She had looked up from Angie's shoulder and was peering up the garden. Somebody was coming.

Through the smoke a shape appeared.

'I'm here,' it said hoarsely.

Jasmine gasped.

'Derek?' I enquired.

It was indeed Derek, out of breath, sweaty and rather crumpled.

'Been looking for you all over Jas. Wanted to surprise you.'

'Now what?' I asked.

Derek went to the table, twisted open a lemonade bottle and took a long swig. Then he turned to address us all.

'I've been a fool,' he said. 'I've known almost from the first moment what I wanted. I even wrote it down in the magic ceremony when we had to say what would make us happy. But, it was hard to break free from what I was. And then with all that übermensch stuff he put in my head, I went back to it. I bought a ticket to Bangkok'

'And did you have a nice time?' I queried, 'The pagodas, the water market…?'

'Jasmine didn't want me to go, said Derek, ignoring me. 'But I said that I had to, because' (here he turned to me) 'I believed what you had told me about the will, and how truly exceptional people broke free from convention and "so called" morality and set off for uncharted waters.'

'Well, yes, that's Nietzsche's idea.' I confirmed.

'Before I left,' said Derek 'Jasmine gave me a book.'

'A book? Jasmine doesn't read books!'

Derek pulled a small paperback from his pocket, and I was astonished and then rather annoyed to see that it was Plato's *The Republic.* It was the one book that I felt necessary to warn the GPs to steer clear of—I had had more than enough trouble with it after Stuart had obtained a copy in America.

'Jasmine!' I said, 'I told you not to read that!'

'Well, I never actually finished it.'

'But I did,' said Derek. 'I read it in one sitting on the flight out. And it set me thinking. Thinking so much that when I got to Bangkok airport I bought another ticket and flew straight back. Back to the girl I love. He pulled the message from his pocket. 'Jasmine, this is what I wrote when we did Hegel's diet. It's the secret that would make me happy.' Jasmine took it, unfolded the paper and read it slowly. Wendy and Angie both peeped over her shoulder and read it too. From their reaction, Derek had obviously written something soppy.

Derek looked imploringly at Jasmine. For a while she continued to stare down at the paper and her face remained impassive, then she looked up and smiled at him. He laughed and smiled happily, perhaps the first really nice smile I had seen Derek ever give. Then they hugged. There was small round of applause from the other Guinea Pigs and the Vicar's wife. I edged closer and politely joined in, looking for my chance. Still gripped in Derek's embrace, the manuscript began to slip gradually from Jasmine's fingers until it flopped to the ground, but before I could reach it Angie quickly scooped it up, and when Jasmine and Derek eventually disengaged she passed it to him.

'What's this?'

'It's his diet book. We're wondering if we should burn it,' Angie explained.

Derek smiled in his more usual rather nasty way, took a firm hold of the manuscript and looked at the fire. I was again anxious—it was so easy to misinterpret *The Republic*.

'I learned two things from Plato on that flight,' said Derek, 'The first is what you called "strong will" is not will at all, it's just desire, and I wasn't being strong by following it like what you said, I was being weak.'

'Well, I was speaking hypothetically in Nietzsche's voice...' I began.

'The second thing I found out,' interrupted Derek, 'was that there are some people, who think that they're philosophers but really they're not.' Derek opened the book to a page he had marked and began to read:

' "a bald little blacksmith fresh out of prison dressed in his best clothes smelling of bath salts... ".'

The passage Derek was reading described the ancient Greek equivalent of someone that we might call a 'yob' or a 'chav' strutting about bathed in aftershave, vainly imagining that he was somehow equipped to engage in philosophy, and I could barely suppress my laughter. It was, of course, a marvellously exact description of Derek himself, with his clumsy efforts to understand the classics. In fact, it encapsulated Derek's problem. He had been trying to engage in philosophy, but basically he couldn't. He was just too bald, too much the ex-con, too covered in aftershave.

'So you've worked it out have you Derek? I asked, 'Who that person sounds like?'

'Yes,' said Derek. 'They're like you.'

There was a long and sinister silence broken only by the malevolent crackling of the fire.

'*I'm* not bald,' I said.

'Let's not get caught up in appearances,' replied Derek. 'The reality is that you're hopelessly out of your depth, have been from the beginning. You know *nothing* about philosophy.'

'Yes I do.'

'No you don't, I looked you up while I was waiting to fly back. You've never written one book on it.'

'But you've got the manuscript to my book right there!'

'You're not in a philosophy department, and in fact your university doesn't even have one.'

'Well it used to.'

'The fact is, you're a fraud, no better than this blacksmith. And not just a fraud, you're a conman. Because you've been conning us, making out that you're this big philosophy expert when you're not, wasting our time, ruining our relationships. And telling us lies.'

'Dialectics.'

Whatever, it's all been deliberate. Setting us up all the way along. Getting Stuart and Wendy to take you on holiday, then leaving Wendy behind.'

'It's hardly my fault that a squirrel bit her.'

'And the diet contract. Angie's still got the bruises. I bet you knew Wendy was coming back, probably tipped the Vicar off too.'

'I did not!'

And the orange buckets. Some gift. Those buckets come in normal and extra-strength. Why did you buy normal?'

'Well, I didn't think...'

'I bet you did. But it was when it came to the Germans you really started. Taking advantage of Jasmine's innocence.'

'I never.'

'Feeding Stuart tapeworms.'

'We've already discussed that before you came and agreed that it was his own fault.'

'And then telling us that story like we were the hero when really we were the baddie, the President.'

'Well, yes, I did do that.'

'So basically you've been messing us about the whole way through.'

'No, Not me. You see philosophy enters a crisis after Nietzsche starts going on and on about the Death of God. It makes philosophers realise that they don't actually know what morality is any longer, and the only alternatives seem to be either to abandon all that they thought they knew since Plato and pursue desires without restraint, or to just give up thinking about it altogether.'

'No need to mess *us* up though.'

'No, I didn't mean to. I thought that when we got to the crisis point, because you *weren't* philosophers, you wouldn't even realise it, so it wouldn't bother you. I mean apart from Jasmine, when I pretended to you that you were übermensch you seemed happy about it.'

'Happy? You made us happy by getting us to imagine that we were a sort of Nazi?'

There was a reproachful silence as the pyre of books sparked and flamed.

'I think,' I said, 'that it is time for me to explain another diet to you.'

Everyone groaned.

'It won't take too long, and although it is based on a kind of post-Marxist philosophy called 'existentialism' that is rather hard to read, you can grasp its essentials very quickly, particularly if you've seen Kirk Douglas in the movie

Spartacus, or even Arnold Schwarznegger in *The Running Man*.'

'Alright,' said Derek, 'You've got five minutes.'

Albert Camus

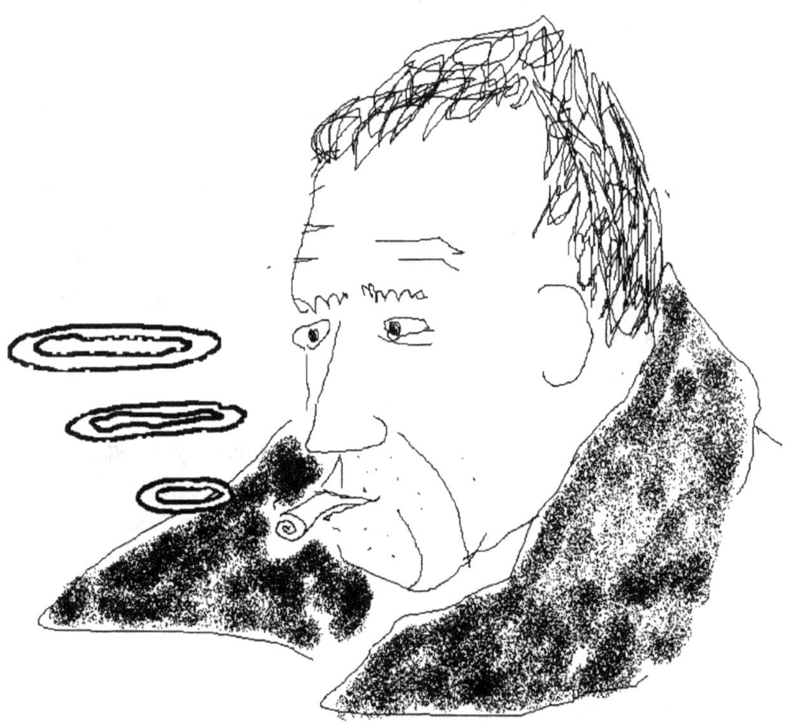

Spartacus and the Fastidious Assassins

' "Everything is pointless"—That, Jasmine, is a *fantastic* insight. I mean it. You've realised that betrayed by Knud and with no island paradise to look forward to, all of our dieting efforts have been meaningless. Well, in philosophical terms that realisation is a huge step forward. If philosophy started with Plato in the fifth century BC it took about 2,300 years before Schopenhauer finally said that with no God and no heaven everything we do is meaningless: "all sound and fury signifying nothing".* And obviously that includes dieting. So the question is, once you *realise* everything is pointless, what do you do about it? It took philosophers another 100 years to work the answer to that one out, and the man who cracked it was a French-Algerian called Albert Camus.

The first thing Camus worked out was what *not* to do. If there is no God, it is a big mistake to go and sit in God's throne, and imagine that you are like Him. That leads to disaster because soon you start to imagine that you know best about everything and that if only other people would only do as you told them, then things would be perfect. Sit on God's throne and you end up believing that if anyone gets in the way of your plans, then you can kill them. Now who does that remind you of?'

The Guinea Pigs pondered that question while I waited, assuming that someone would come up with a name like Stalin, or Hitler, or Knudson. Instead Angie said:

'You: it sounds like you Peter. You don't kill us, but you're a know-it-all and if we'd done your diets properly you think we'd be perfect.'

There was a short silence while the fire crackled malevolently a bit, but by now I was starting to get used to these kinds of accusations and took it in my stride.

'Well, you are sort of right Angie, because that is certainly the attitude of some of the diet gurus whose books you've been burning. But although I might seem like a guru to you, I'm not, and I never have been. For one thing, I've read

* A quotation from *Macbeth* by Shakespeare.

Camus, so I knew when I set out to teach you these diets that there would be no magic formula, and that quite probably everything would go wrong. I admit that I was—and am—excited about the bucket diet. But once you stopped using your buckets, I thought that if *that* didn't work, then the Four Germans were unlikely to help, and you'd all end up as overweight as ever.'

As I said this, I noticed again that Angie was *not* actually as overweight as she had been before and that Jasmine too was somewhat slimmer. But I did not let this fact interrupt the flow of logic.

'So,' I concluded, 'it's actually all been just as pointless for me as it has been for you. And when you ask "why put us through all that?" *I've* been through it too. I've been betrayed by Knudson as much as you have. But it is not just that, because I have also known, from the very start, that it was pointless. But I've done it anyway. And why? Because of Camus, and what he said about the Spartacus Rebellion.

'We started our diets by looking in the mirror and thinking about ourselves and laughing about it. Well when Spartacus thought about himself he realised that something was wrong and it was no laughing matter. It was not that anything *looked* wrong. Spartacus was a gladiator so we can be pretty certain that he had a superb iron stomach and was generally in great shape. But Spartacus was also a slave, and *that* was wrong. Now, it may appear that being a slave is a very different problem to being overweight, but in fact they are remarkably similar. Spartacus was a slave to the Romans, while someone who is overweight is a slave to food. But this is not food in the old fashioned sense of the word. Let's go back to Karl Marx for a minute. Whatever you think of Marx, he makes it obvious that the modern food to which people are enslaved is not from their local farmer, but is produced by gigantic multinational conglomerates, with their incessant advertising-propaganda and ubiquitous supermarkets, 'convenience' stores, fast-food restaurants and snack machines.

'Spartacus, then, was up against a mighty empire, and when you try and break free of your slavery to food, so are you. And if you fight against a huge and powerful enemy, one thing is pretty much certain: you are going to lose. Spartacus must have known that if he escaped and started out on a campaign against the might of Rome, he would lose. But he tried anyway. With about forty other gladiators he broke free and took to the mountains. He rebelled, *even though it was pointless*.

'Then an amazing thing happened. Spartacus's rebellion began to succeed. His little band of followers turned into a vast army of thousands of slaves. They won a series of stunning victories until finally they arrived at the very gates of Rome.

'Spartacus looked down from a hill at the city spread helplessly below him and *he turned away*. He ordered his army not to attack, but to retreat.

'Why? Why, when victory was so close, did Spartacus seem to give up? Spartacus had realised that he did not *want* to win, not if it meant being *just like them*. For if he had captured Rome he would have been enthroned as emperor, treated as a god, his enemies enslaved and everything as bad as it was before. So he retreated, back the way he had come searching, Camus says, for the pure roots of his rebellion, until the Roman army caught up with him and his army and killed them all.

'So what is the rebel diet? It is a diet that whenever it starts to succeed, then starts to fail. On the rebel diet, when you really start to lose significant weight you react like Spartacus. You realise that if you finally succeed in losing weight and looking great *you will become one of them*, one of the enemy, the oppressors. Your superb body will become a walking insult to the group you once belonged to, the food-slaves who remain overweight. Your very transformation will remind them of their slavery to food, you will seem to lord it over them. And you yourself will probably start to behave differently towards them, letting them know that you are no longer their equal but their superior. You will become condescending, narcissistic and arrogant. You will become like the A team.

'It is because you sense this that when your diet is on the brink of success you start overeating again. At the very point when your fat begins rapidly to vanish you turn your back on your diet. You cannot bring yourself to finally triumph over food slavery until everyone is free. It is your solidarity with them, your fellow overweightees—if I may put it that way—that keeps your weight oscillating.

'At the beginning of the twentieth century anarchist bands in Russia were busy murdering people because they were rich or because they worked for the state. Camus approved. He called these anarchists the fastidious assassins. To be fastidious usually means to be choosy about your food, but the fastidious assassins were choosy about who they killed. In an unjust world they thought (1) it was necessary to murder people, but it was also (2) inexcusable. So they were always very careful about murdering only those people that they thought really deserved it and then they allowed themselves to get caught afterwards. Although not *exactly* the same, you are trapped in a similar dilemma with your diet: you realise (1) that you must diet and at the same time (2) that you must not. So your weight goes up and down as you battle first against being overweight and then against the power structure that enslaves millions of others into being overweight. If this diet ever succeeded it would be a sell-out to the enemy. The purpose, the heroism and, yes, the glamour of the rebel diet is that it will fail.'

I paused, then turned to Derek.

'Derek,' I said, 'You were always a bit of a rebel, and I think Jasmine's got the making of a rebel too. And Stuart, you're a wonderful rebel, the Che Guevara of dieting! Look at how you've tried one diet after another, and none of them have worked at all. That's brilliant! Those failures aren't pointless; they're the very thing that makes life worth living. You Guinea Pigs, guys, are an inspiration.'

There was another silence at this while the fire flickered doubtfully. It was not quite the same sort of silence that I had heard when I told them that being fat was their own fault. That had been the shocked silence of a home truth. This was a more suspicious sort of silence, a silence in which the Guinea Pigs seemed to feel that they had just been taken in by some verbal trickery, without quite knowing how. They looked at each other, communicating with cheeks and eyebrows and shoulder shrugs. Finally Derek spoke up.

'OK, I sort of get it. A rebel knows he'll lose because he's up against a whole system. Like Robin Hood against the Sheriff of Nottingham. He knows they'll get him in the end because they've got the money and the castles. And a diet-rebel knows he'll lose too but tries anyway, and it's good just to try.'

'Exactly Derek,' I said, 'and, if I may say so, I think that Jasmine makes a lovely Maid Marion.'

Jasmine rolled her eyes. 'Oh give him his thing back,' she said.

Somewhat begrudgingly Derek held out the manuscript. But before I could take it, the Vicar's wife stepped between us and deftly removed it from his grasp.

The Rebel Diet in a Nutshell

Diet even though it won't work.

Sources

A. Camus, *The Rebel*

Plato, *Republic*

Chapter 11
The God Diet

This chapter is shorter and a bit different from the others.

God

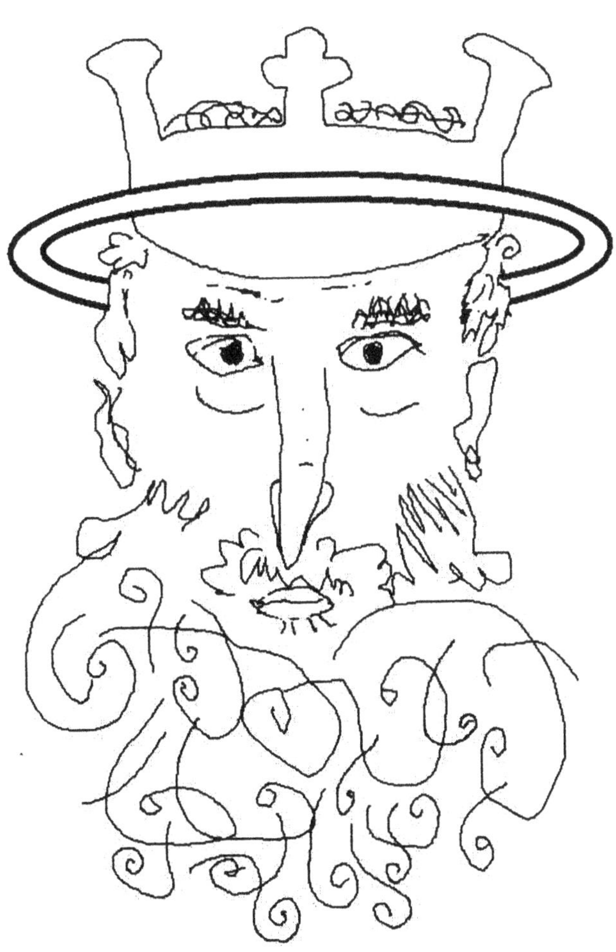

'Edna? Why do *you* want to burn it? You're not even a Guinea Pig.'

I am afraid I sounded irritated, but seemed quite unfair that the Vicar's wife who had only been in the meetings at all when she was hovering around with the teapots and the cakes, should be yet another accuser.

Don't worry Peter, I don't want to burn your book, I want to add something to it. You have been writing me letters. Well, I have written one to you.'

The Vicar's wife passed me a neatly folded sheet of paper. This is what it said.

Dear Peter,
Making your group cakes and things has not really been out of goodness—more curiosity. I was interested in what you were doing, and I wanted to listen in. Perhaps I should have admitted that and joined the group. But I was not really sure that I would have fitted in because I am not overweight. Still, I have heard enough to know that you have been talking about all these philosophers, and they all have diets that you try, and then they don't work properly. And so the question is: why not?

I think I know the answer: Philosophy only makes sense if you believe in God. And the philosophers you have chosen, most of them at least, do not. They are sometimes quite arrogant about this, as if they can explain the whole of human history and human nature without any reference to God at all, unless it is to insult him. Well I do not think that you can do that. Any philosopher who tries to explain the world without God will fail, and this means that their diets will fail too.

So to go on a diet you must first believe in God. Then you need to think about how your way of understanding God is related to going on a diet. In Christianity, dieting is related to self control and resisting temptation. It is about not being greedy and following your inner conscience rather for being out for all you can get. But every major religion , I think, says something similar, And they all encourage you to diet. Muslims practice fasting over Ramadan. Jews have rules about food preparation and prohibited food combinations. Christians fast for lent. Religions also impose diets by prohibiting certain foods altogether. Muslims will not eat pork. Hindus have sacred cows. Shinto priests only eat birds and rabbits. Buddhists are vegetarian. In the Old Testament there are all kinds of rather rigid rules that now, I admit, sound a bit silly, but were then a way of expressing an awareness of God as he was understood at the time. In Leviticus 11, there is a long list of animals that you are allowed to eat (such as cows, sheep and beetles) and others that you are not (such as cuckoos, bats and tortoises). One might even say that the whole history of religion has been an extended argument over what to eat and when to eat it.

So how would I diet as a Christian? The answer is simple. If I wanted to go on a diet I would pray to God, and part of my prayer would be to lose weight.

This might sounds rather selfish. You pray for other people, and even when you pray for yourself, it is so that, somehow you can be a better person towards others. So try not to be selfish about it: pray to lose weight on behalf of others. Perhaps by losing weight you can be more pleasing to your spouse, or better able to play with children, or a better role model, or anything, I am not sure. If you really believe that by losing weight you can better help others, then God will give you the strength to lose weight.

Now imagine this. You pray to lose weight, and you know in your mind that you are meant to be praying for other people, or so that you can be a better person for other people. But you also know in your heart that the main reason you want to lose weight so that you can show off being slim in front of your friends, or something selfish like that. What do you do? After all, there is no point trying to fool God, he will know what you really think just as well as you do. Not bother? No. I think that you should go ahead and pray anyway. Because we all have mixed motives, we feel more than one thing. And somewhere in all of us is a love for others. When you pray, even if you do so mostly for selfish reasons, there will be a little bit of that love mixed in. And God will help to connect you with that little bit, help to make it grow. And the more you pray, the more it will grow. So that is my advice. Pray to lose weight, not for yourself but for other people.

Yours Edna

PS I forgive you for being rude about my biscuits.

So there it is. When I read it out the Guinea Pigs seemed to like it, but maybe they were just being polite. It was slightly irritating that the Vicar's wife herself was so slim, as though this was an advert for the efficacy of prayer, but if you take this line of reasoning you will end up taking cocaine in the hope that you will come to look like Kate Moss. Needless to add, I thought the diet was absurd. Someone who still believes in Noah's Ark is hardly going to add anything to the canon of philosophy. However, the fire was still burning brightly, so I thought it best to be conciliatory.

'What a beautiful letter Edna. I promise to put it in the book. Now *please* can I have my manuscript back?'

'No Peter. I *would* give it you back, but I think Angie wants a word with you first.' And with that the Vicar's wife passed my manuscript to Angie.

The God Diet in a Nutshell
Pray.

Chapter 12
The Love Diet

which explains how to lose weight by climbing the ladder of love.

Alcibiades

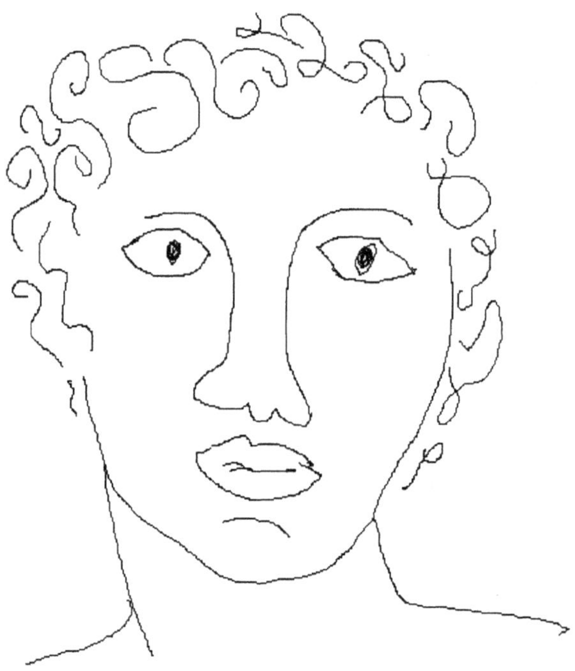

'You said I was special,' said Angie, rolling up my manuscript and pointing it at me accusingly, 'special and unique and superior with an "incandescent inner-beauty." You said all that, I thought, only to me. But now I find that you were saying exactly the same thing to everyone.'

'Well, not *exactly* the same thing.'

Did you tell Jasmine that she was special and beautiful?'

'Well, metaphorically…' I began.

'Yes,' cut in Jasmine bluntly.

'And you even said something like that to Stuart and Derek?'

'He said I had a "luminous inner-handsomeness",' affirmed Derek.

'And I look like a Greek God,' said Stuart in a smug tone that suggested that he had still not wholly grasped that, in fact, he did not.

'So,' pointed out Angie, 'you hadn't really singled me out when you were saying those sweet things just to me; you were betraying me.'

'Well, dialectically speaking I was…'

'Dialectically speaking you were lying. You were betraying us all, but you hurt me most. Because Stuart has Wendy to tell him nice things,' Angie continued.

'And I do think he looks like a Greek God,' broke in Wendy loyally. 'He looks like Bacchus.'*

'And now Jasmine has Derek,' continued Angie.

'Jasmine looks like a God too, she looks like Diana,'** said Derek.

---

* Curious readers may wish to look up Rubens' painting of Bacchus who, at least as portrayed in this picture, does indeed bear a striking resemblance to Stuart.

** Diana Goddess of the Hunt is the subject of hundreds of paintings and sculptures. The best sculpture, strikingly erotic, is on a fountain in a courtyard at the University of Illinois where I gained my PhD. People would eat their lunch around the fountain, but I always found Diana so diverting that I could never really concentrate on my sandwiches. From this experience I began to understand Plato's love diet.

Jasmine flushed pink, 'Well that bulimia diet did work a bit, sort of,' she said modestly.

'But I,' said Angie 'I have no one.'

There was a silence as the fire crackled sadly.

'Angie,' I said, 'I'm sorry, truly sorry, if you think I betrayed you. But I need to explain something else, something very important about the origins of western philosophy. I haven't told you yet but I always meant to tell you.'

'What?'

'It all started, philosophy started, with a love affair that went badly wrong. Do you remember that the diet of pigs was written down by Plato, but was in the voice of Socrates? Well, when Plato was a young man he was in love with Socrates.'

'And that was the failed affair?'

'No. Lots of young men were in love with Socrates, even though he was old and ugly. But he never took any notice of them. Except for one. There was a man called Alcibiades who was wildly attractive and exceptionally talented. Socrates noticed him and the pair soon became inseparable.'

The Ladder of Love

Because of his intelligence, charisma, audacity and intense, passionate nature, Alcibiades was destined for a great future. But his character was on a knife-edge, and if it tipped the wrong way, the same qualities that could make him great would make him terrible. A knife-edge, however, is not quite the right metaphor. Alcibiades was actually on a ladder, the ladder of love, and Socrates wanted to make sure that he went up it and not down.

The steps on the ladder are as follows.

The Ladder of Love

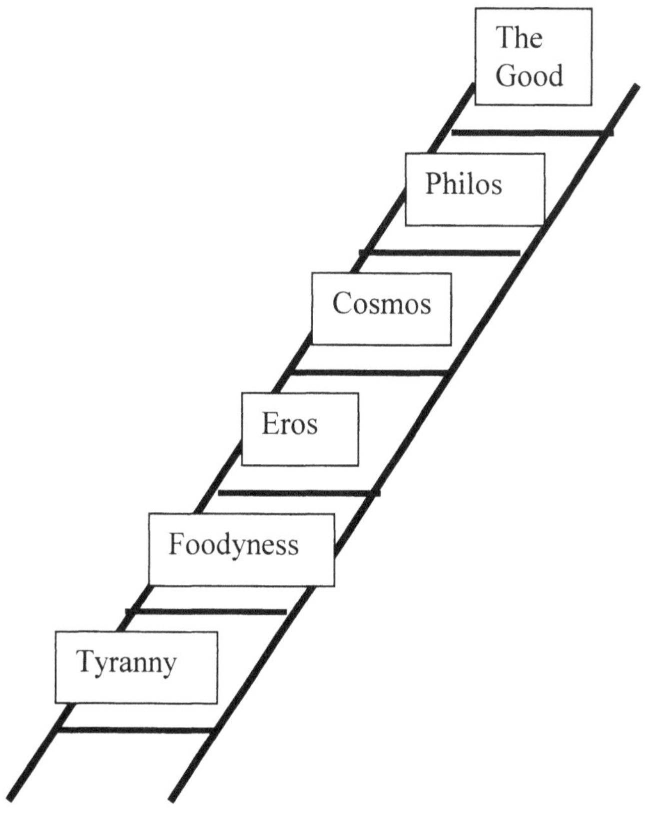

Step 1 At the very base of the ladder is tyranny: meaning selfish lust and treating other people as objects for your own gratification.

Step 2 The next step up is foodyness (or *adephagia* the spirit of gluttony). This is the love of food and drink and its enjoyment. On this step you treat the food you love as an object for your gratification, but at least it *is* an object: so that's a step up the ladder!

Step 3 is eros or sexual love. Erotic love is a yearning for someone you love to love you back, physically. When you feel eros you realise that your beloved is beautiful and want to unite yourself with this beauty.

Step 4 is cosmos where you feel a yearning for nature and love the beauty of the world and of the universe.

Step 5 Philos (as in philosophy) is when you bring the natural and human worlds together love them both and want to understand them.

Step 6 At the top of the ladder is love of the good, of doing right, acting morally.

Socrates was at the top of the ladder, even above philosophy, because he loved the good, and Alcibiades was on the third step, eros, because he had a powerful erotic desire for Socrates. Socrates was worried that Alcibiades might slip down the ladder into tyrannical lust, and was trying instead to get him to climb *up* the ladder. So he told Alcibiades about the cosmos, explaining things like how thunder and lightning were natural phenomena and not the gods in a bad mood. Meanwhile, Alcibiades was trying to get Socrates to climb *down* the ladder to have an erotic relationship with him. He did this, not very subtly, by contriving to share a bed with Socrates and arranging nude wrestling bouts together and things like that.

But, as I say, it all went horribly wrong.

It happened by accident almost. With all the things Socrates was telling him about the cosmos and philosophy Alcibiades stopped believing in God, or at least, he stopped believing in the Greek gods. The Greeks had numerous rituals and rules about their gods, ones that they took very seriously. One ritual involved lots of virgin girls in a mysterious temple ceremony. And one rule was that every house had to have standing at its gates a stature, called a Hermes statue of a male torso, *with all the bits*. After all the things Socrates had explained to him, it was only natural that Alcibiades saw the funny side of this. Hardly surprising, therefore, that one evening he and some of his friends dressed in women's clothing and pretended to enact the secret ceremony of the virgin girls. Then, in the middle of the night, they went running through the streets stopping at the gates of every house to break off a *bit* of its Hermes stature.

I will leave you to guess *which* bit they broke off.

In the morning the Athenian citizens were outraged. Their statues all had bits broken off them and dreadful rumours were circulating about young men dressed in women's clothing mocking the sacred ceremony of the virgins.

Alcibiades and his friends were wealthy aristocrats so in normal times a little escapade like this would all have been smoothed over. Some hapless slave would have been framed to take the blame and that would have been that. But the times were not normal. Athens was at war with Sparta and Alcibiades had been made a general and put in charge of a fleet of ships that were about to sail and engage the enemy. And before anything had been sorted out, Alcibiades embarked on this expedition, leaving the Athenians behind to seethe over their insulted virgins and emasculated statues. What made things worse was that if Alcibiades won the battle and returned victorious, they could hardly start making a fuss about it *then*. So they sent out a messenger, ordering Alcibiades to come back at once to stand trial.

It must have seemed absurdly vindictive and petty to Alcibiades, voyaging to battle, to be told to return to Athens to account for a bit of horseplay. Nonetheless he told that messenger that of course he would come. But he didn't. Instead he slipped away and went over to Sparta.

Alcibiades met the Spartan king and told him of a weakness in the walls around Athens. The excited king took his army and rushed to attack this weak spot, leaving Alcibiades behind with the queen. Alcibiades made her pregnant.

Alcibiades slipped away from Sparta and made his way back to Athens, where they had managed to fend off the attack. He frankly admitted what he had done and said that the verve and audacity he had shown in betraying them was exactly why the Athenians needed him if they wanted to win the war. So they took him back and kept him as a general. But in the end, they still lost.

Alcibiades slipped away to an island, but the Athenians caught up with him and had him assassinated. Then they looked around for who else to blame, and turned on his lover, Socrates.

So Socrates was put on trial for 'corrupting the youth of Athens' (meaning Alcibiades); teaching about the natural world and the cosmos; teaching philosophy—which his accusers said was no better than sophistry, and not believing in the gods. He was convicted and sentenced to die by drinking poisonous hemlock.

Plato watched the trial. Horrified at the sentence he joined a conspiracy to bribe the guards so that Socrates could escape—but Socrates refused to escape. And Plato was also there when Socrates drank the poison.

Socrates had never written things down, he was only concerned with being good. So after the execution of the man he loved, Plato dedicated the rest of his life to recording the things that Socrates had said in his dialogues. And that is how western philosophy started.

The Love Delta

To relate the story of Alcibiades to dieting we are going to add artistry to the ladder of love, and then turn the whole ladder into a love delta. Love is a river that flows through us all. But as we grow up, this love breaks up into lots of smaller rivers that fan out like a delta.

Everyone has this river flowing through them, but it flows at different strengths. Some people, like Alcibiades, have a great flood of love flowing through them, for others it is a mere trickle. And as this river of love reaches the delta it flows at different rates through different channels. For Alcibiades most of his river of love flowed through the eros channel. If you are overweight then too much of your river of love is flowing through the foodyness channel. Now at one level, this is exciting, because the more overweight you are, the more love that there is flowing through you. If you are really obese, then you actually have loads of love, probably

The Love Delta

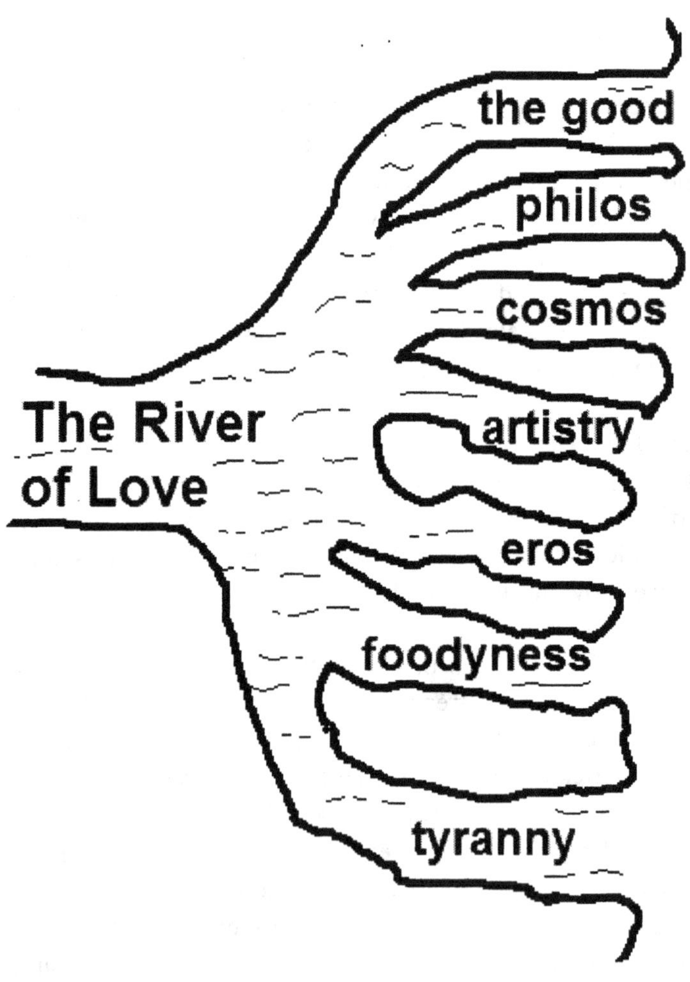

much more than most people! The problem, of course, is that this love, or most of it, is flowing down *the wrong channel.* The solution, equally obvious, is to divert the flow of love away from the foodyness channel and send it down a different channel (or channels) instead.

Which channel should we choose to divert the flow of love? Let's start by ruling out tyranny. It is better by far to be fat and nice to other people than to be a great looking tyrant. And let's be realistic and cut out 'the good' too. While it would undoubtedly solve your weight problem if you could spend your time loving the good, it is probably aiming too high. That leaves four channels: philos, cosmos, artistry and eros. You have to ask: which of these will work for you.

Philos Has reading this book left you thirsting for more philosophy? If so you may be able to divert your river of love down the philos channel.

But what if philosophy leaves you cold? Then you might try:

Cosmos The cosmos we live in can drive people wild with passion. Some gaze at the stars, others collect plankton in a stocking and examine it under a microscope. If that kind of thing inspires you then go for it! The more you engage with nature, the more you will lose weight.

Artistry Do you love music, painting drama, things like that? If you really love them, then develop your passion and you can send the flow of love down the artistry artery.

At this point you might be thinking: 'Yes, I am interested enough in philosophy, and nature, and the arts. But I'm not sure that I exactly 'love' them, not like I love my partner/spouse—or at least the person I *wish* was my partner etc. If that is what you are thinking, well done! It gets right to the heart of the love diet because you have to *literally* love these things for the love diet to work. And if you don't love them already, at least a little bit, then it is going to be very hard, and probably unrealistic to start to love them from scratch. It is much easier to divert more of the river of love down a channel that is already flowing than to dig a whole new channel. So before we make a failed effort, we have to try and see if any of these channels already have love-water flowing through them. OK. How?

Here is a simple test to see whether you do love them—a test that I began immediately with the Guinea Pigs once they understood what was required of them.

A Simple Test

This test is, as I say, very simple. But it is also time consuming. It is going to require at least three and perhaps four blocks of time. And it might feel a bit frustrating because although we are near the end of the book, it is better if you do the test without reading ahead.

OK. First, *for those readers who are in a relationship*, I want you to have an erotic lovemaking session with your partner lasting 2 ½ to 3 hours. For those who are not in a relationship, don't worry, you can simply keep on reading and do the other tests.

Lovemaking over? OK. Now choose one of the things that you at least quite enjoy doing: say reading a book of philosophy (philos), or bird watching (cosmos), or playing a musical instrument (artistry). The test is this: *Go and do it* for between 2 ½ and 3 hours. Set this time aside so that you can do whatever you are doing without interruption, so that you can do it constantly.

Now try out an activity that you might love from the other two categories too. Each one needs a separate 2 ½-3 hour block of time, uninterrupted time.

All done? OK. How are we going to interpret these tests? By answering this question:

Whatever it was you did, before the task in hand was finished did you take a break for a bit and have something to eat (perhaps a snack like a sandwich or a cup of tea and a slice of cake)?

Philos: Yes/No
Cosmos: Yes/No
Artistry: Yes/No

If you answered yes then *you do not love what you do*. You might still enjoy it greatly, but you do not actually love it.

How do I know this? Because of eros. No one, while having erotic sex, takes a break for sandwich *half way through.* Neither, incidentally would they rush to finish early so as to leave time for a good nosh. I do not even need to ask *that* question.

It is helpful for people who are in relationships to actually try this out for themselves to confirm it. But if you are not in a relationship, then you may well not need to confirm it, because you may be *hopelessly in love*. And if you imagine a fairy godmother waving a wand that allowed you to spend a magical 2 ½ to 3 hours in an erotic encounter with your beloved, you would hardly want to waste this time eating sandwiches together, or even ice cream. In fact, if you are *hopelessly* in love, from a dieting perspective this is very good news because it sends your love river gushing down the eros channel. Having an active sex life with your partner also helps channel eros, but unfortunately it is liable to become less effective in the long term—from a purely statistical point of view this is obvious for otherwise everyone who leads a full married life would be slim, and needless to say they are not. With sexual fulfilment there is a gradual slackening of the flow of eros as the river of love slowly begins to stagnate. Eventually there comes a time when faced with the choice between a daytime romp and a meal, you and your partner choose the meal *even though you are not particularly hungry*, and the foodyness channel starts to flow again. But as long as you maintain a hopeless, yearning, unrequited love, there is no danger of this; it's the ideal method of losing weight and looking great!

Conversation with Angie

Angie and I were alone by the fire. The rather harsh atmosphere had lightened when I had explained the love diet. The Guinea Pigs had particularly liked the idea that the more overweight you were, the deeper the love river coursing though your body. So when I proposed that they take the simple test, Derek and Jasmine had immediately gone off to give it a try, and after Stuart had whispered something about making love to a Greek God, he and Wendy had slipped away too. The Vicar's wife had also tactfully withdrawn.

Angie, however, still had hold of my manuscript.

'Peter, can I ask you questions that you promise to answer honestly?'

'Alright.'

'Do you think that it is true that fatter people have more love flowing through them?'

'Well not literally, but dialectically. I mean, if it was literally true that Stuart, Derek and Jasmine had a huge flood of love flowing through them, then I wouldn't have told then they were übermensch, because then they might have got up to some mischief like Alcibiades did. But I knew that actually they were pretty harmless. So it was another dialectical way of encouraging them to do something with their lives.'

'Encouraging us to get off the foodyness step on the ladder of love, and get on to another step?'

Yes. I know it didn't work very well, but...'

'It *did* work Peter. It worked on *me*. I moved. I moved up the ladder.'

'What do you mean?'

Before Angie could answer her phone beeped and the question was left hanging in the air.

'It's just a text message from Wendy asking if I can bring up a few buns,' explained Angie as she put my manuscript under her arm, gathered some pastries on a plate and went inside the house.

I was left to wonder. I was starting to feel bad about using dialectics on the Guinea Pigs. I wished I could start again and use logic instead. Perhaps it might have worked better. And I was feeling other things as well. About Angie, about our conversations together, how I had enjoyed them. The fun we'd had on the überdiet, the way in which she had been so abrasive and yet so honest in revealing intimate details of her metabolism in the bucket diet. And now all the trust had gone between us. It was the Four Germans' fault, I thought. Hegel, Marx, Schopenahauer and Nietzsche: all their nasty ideas had got in the way of our relationship. No, I realised with shock. It *wasn't* their fault. They had not *made* me do what I had done. It was *my* fault.

Angie came back.

'Peter, answer honestly again, where do you think that *you* are on the ladder of love?'

'Well,' I said modestly, 'I hardly like to say. 'I think, I mean…'

'Do you think you are up there with Socrates, right up at the top?'

'Well. Ha ha. I mean even Plato wasn't as high as *that*, he loved philos so, I suppose, well, as a fellow philosopher …'

'I see. You think you're on the philos step. Shall I tell you where I think you are?'

'Where?'

'I think you're right down at the bottom, on tyranny.'

Another nasty allegation.

'Tyranny? Why?'

'Because that's how you've been treating us Guinea Pigs: as objects to play around with, to manipulate, to lie to, just like a tyrant. And you've been enjoying it.'

'That's not true Angie.'

'I think it is and that's why this should go in the fire. But I can't do it. Take the stupid thing back.'

I took the manuscript back and looked at it doubtfully.

Angie started to walk away.

'Angela!' I called. 'Wait!'

She kept walking.

'Please Angie!'

She turned. 'What?'

'I love you.'

Angie tossed her head.

I threw the manuscript on the fire. I realised that was going to have to rewrite quite a lot of it anyway.

***

Three hours later, Angie and I wandered out of the woods and back into the garden. The fire had died down, but some of the cakes were still there and we both felt surprisingly hungry. Derek and Jasmine, it would seem, were going to marry. Angie had told me that Derek's note as to what would make him happy had simply said 'Marry Jasmine'. And Angie and I had decided that we may as well get married too. We neither of us were getting any younger and Angie wanted to see if we could arrange a double wedding. We both agreed that it would be an excellent idea for us to be married by the Vicar and hold the reception in the church hall (with Edna making the wedding cake). I was curious about what the Vicar would say to this proposal, and hoped that he would accept it with a truly Christian grace if not outright joy. But if he didn't, I had the feeling that as a parishioner baptised into the Church of England, I was within my rights to *demand* that he marry us, so in a way I was also hoping that he would try and refuse.

'Do you know Angie, I think there's a fascinating parallel in all this.'

'Go on?'

'Fyodor Dostoyevsky, he's a novelist from Russia. Well, in his most famous book, *Crime and Punishment*, a man called Raskolnikov chops up two ladies with an axe.

'Oh. That doesn't sound very philosophical.'

'No, but afterwards, he confesses to it, because he's redeemed by the love of a prostitute.'

'So?'

'Well, don't you see? I'm a bit like Raskolnikov. And you're sort of like Sofia, the prostitute.

'Charming!'

'Not *literally* of course. I mean, obviously you're not, and I didn't actually murder any of you either. But *philosophically* this is really interesting. In fact, I think it could be the start of a whole new diet ...'

'Oh shut up!' said Angie.

I shut up. Stuart and Wendy were coming outside. They were both smiling. Derek had sent a text message that he and Jasmine needed a bit longer.

The Love Diet in a Nutshell

Fall in love, preferably hopelessly.

Sources

Aristophanes, *Clouds*
Plato *Apology*
Plato *Crito*
Plato *Phaedo*
Plato *Republic*
Plato *Symposium*
Thucidides, *History of the Peloponnesian War*

Postscript
Philosophy and Desire

Our diets have now been set out. You have twelve of them at least to choose from, more if you count some of the variations within each chapter. And I wish you best of luck with them. None of these diets have been simply made up, but neither, with one or two exceptions, can you find them explicitly laid down; they have been *extrapolated* from philosophical works.

Philosophers rarely talk directly about dieting. Rather, they talk more generally about our desires, including our desire for food, but also for power, sex, money, fame. At a personal level they aim to help us to work out what to do with these desires. And at a social or political level they help us to understand how these desires play out and shape our society and our government. This effort to come to terms with desire underpins what philosophers tell us about how we should live our lives, about what is going on in the world, about the nature of men and of women, about war and peace. I have not said much about all this as I have wanted to concentrate on drawing out the implications for dieting. But now that the story is over and our characters—let us hope—are all living happily ever after, it might be of interest to sketch the broad outlines of the more general philosophical investigation into desire.

Limited and Unlimited Desire

Aristophanes described how the world was once populated by people who were hermaphrodites and who looked like this:

Aristophanes' Hermaphrodite: Before

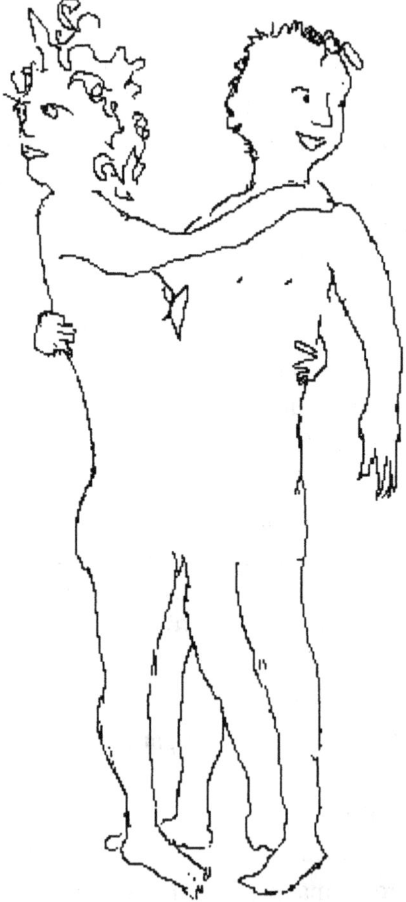

They had two heads and four arms and legs. But they annoyed one of the gods, who chopped them in half, drew the skin together over the wound and twisted their heads around. So now we look like this:

Aristophanes' Hermaphrodite: After

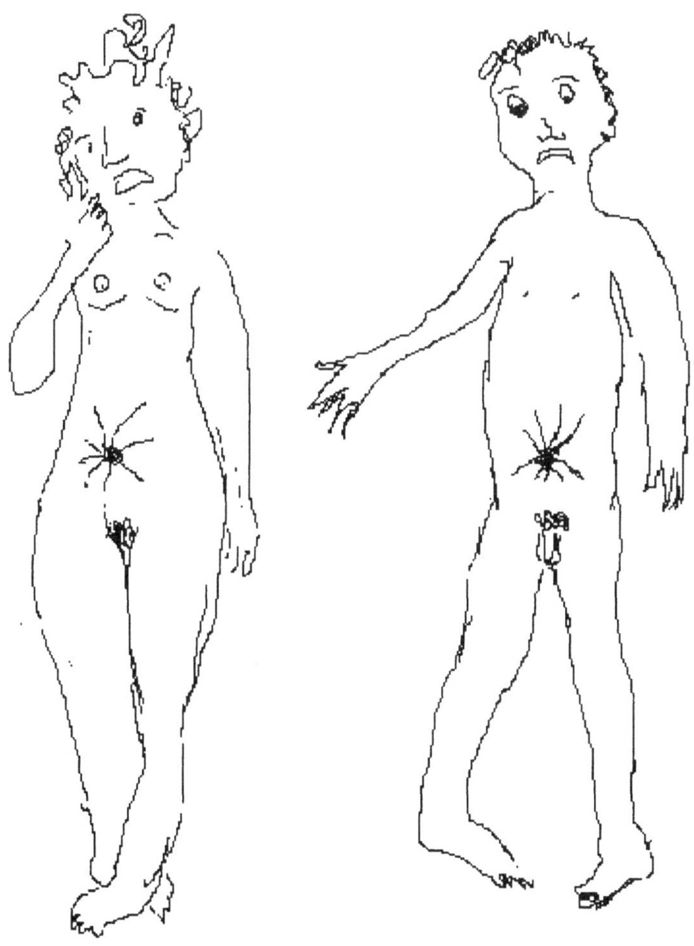

And ever since we have been trying to reunite with our other half. Our love, or desire for a mate, is the feeling that something is missing, something lacking. Desire for a partner is a search to become complete. When we find a mate and regain this sense of completeness our searching desire stops, to be replaced by a settled happiness, or *eudaimon*. So the type of desire described by Aristophanes can be satisfied, it has a goal, it comes to an end.

But there is also a second kind of desire, one that is never satisfied, an insatiable desire. Socrates (who was friendly with Aristophanes) described this desire as being like a greedy seagull, eating and pooing at the same time.

Socrates' Seagull

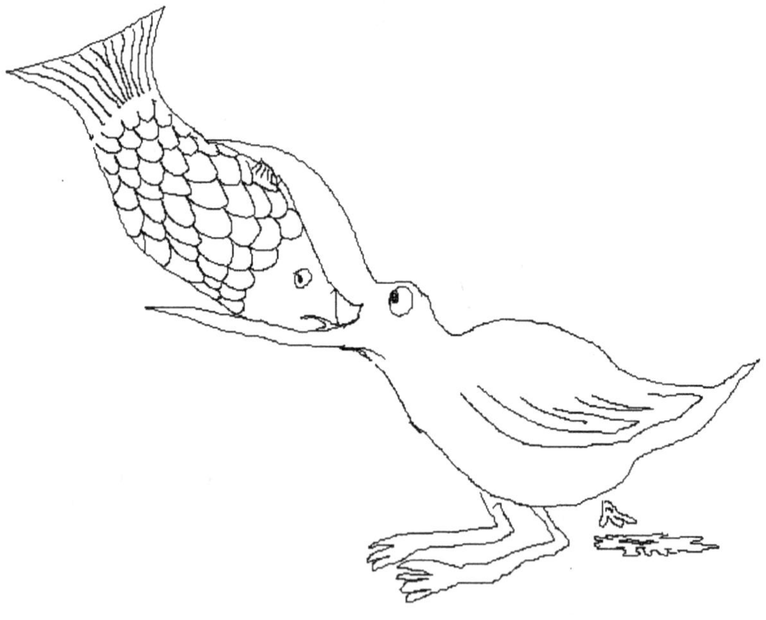

For people who feel they need to diet, it is likely that their attitude to food is, to some extent at least, akin to the unlimited desire of Socrates' seagull. If their diet is to succeed, they must transform this desire into a limited desire, the desire to be complete. But the conflict between these two forms of desires is not just played out within someone attempting to go on a diet, it runs through our entire society. The troublemakers are the voracious seagulls, bringing grief to the rest. And when they become powerful, the seagulls not only cause trouble, but demand that everyone else should be *grateful* to them. Certainly they expect to be paid unlimited amounts of money. They claim to be the wealth creators, the go-getters, the people you need if society is not to stagnate. And this propaganda is squawked so incessantly from every rooftop that many non-seagull people actually believe it.

So much for the way we live now. Let us go back to Hobbes.

Two thousand years after Socrates and Aristophanes distinguished limited and unlimited desire, Hobbes drew a second important distinction between two types of power. One form of power means something very closely akin to 'ability' or 'capacity': our power is our ability to do something, like paint a picture or ride a bike. The second kind of power is power over other people, the power to control them, to boss them around and get them to do things at your behest.

If we put the two forms of power and desire together we end up with four possibilities.

Someone who does not develop their abilities very much because they are satisfied with modest achievements, has the attitude of a jogger. A jogger is not totally inactive, but neither do they put that much effort into their running (nothing wrong with that).

POWER AND DESIRE		Desire:	
		limited	**unlimited**
Power as:	**ability**	jogger	athlete
	control of other people	egalitarian	tyrant

Someone who desires to develop their abilities without limit has the attitude of an athlete: they are always trying to push at the boundaries of what they can do, they make dedicated and concerted efforts to extend their capacities.

Someone who does not desire much power over others quickly comes to a very sensible view: let us all have about the same amount of power and the same rights: they adopt an attitude of live and let live, they are egalitarian.

By contrast, someone who pursues a desire for unlimited power over others is a would-be tyrant.

People do not fit neatly into any one box. Sometimes they may be like joggers, sometimes athletes, sometimes egalitarian and sometimes tyrannical. Nor is it always obvious into which box any activity should go. If someone spends many hours each day watching TV, does this indicate their very limited ambition to develop their own abilities, or does it indicate their insatiable appetite for more TV, fed by ever more channels? So things are more complex than the boxes might suggest, but still they provide a basic framework, a starting point to try and understand the predicament we are in.

The propaganda of the tyrants (for our seagulls have now become tyrants) is to present their desires as akin to the desires of the athlete, to suggest that their drive has given them pre-eminent abilities, whereas in fact it represents only their insatiable greed. Where this type of propaganda holds sway, people who are not powerful (even if they would like to be) are encouraged to develop other forms of insatiable greed, including greed for food. The philosophy of dieting seeks to counter this propaganda. It tries to identify other ways of thinking, ones that will place limits on our less elevated desires, including the desire for more food, either by encouraging us to be more ambitious in developing other better desires, or by appealing directly to our reason.

What puts a limit on our desire? Plato's response was that out desire was kept in check by our reason. But what is 'reason'? I think it is somehow connected to our conscience, but the question is not so easy to answer, and perhaps this explains why a rather glib get-out response from Hume is so famous. According to Hume 'Reason is the instrument of the passions.' This may sound innocent but it is not, because it destroys any idea that reason can act as a counterweight to our desires. We are, says Hume, stuck with our desires, and all our reason does is calculate how best we can pursue them.

The idea that we have no reason independent of our desire is tied to a second idea developed by Hobbes and Baruch Spinoza and popularised by Hume: that we have no free will, meaning that we do not really choose to do anything, but rather every aspect of our behaviour is determined by cause and effect. If, for example, we could analyse the chain of cause and effect sufficiently, we could be no more said to 'choose' to eat a chocolate biscuit than a block of ice could be said to 'choose' to melt in warm sunshine. This idea is so absurd that it is not worth arguing over but the curious fact remains that many philosophers who ought to have known better have been influenced by it to one degree or another.

The philosophical denial of our distinct capacity to reason and to act with free will allowed the idea that Socrates had been arguing *against* more than two thousand years earlier with his seagull metaphor to re-establish itself. Philosophers began to believe that desire was a natural, an inevitable and only state of being, and that, furthermore, the more desire we had the better, so that intense desire was also good. A belief of this sort underlies Hegel's notion that a 'world historical individual' is justified in going round killing people, but the idea really reaches its nadir with Nietzsche.

Nietzsche argues that we do not have free will, but only either strong will (akin to unlimited desire) or weak will (akin to limited desire). He extols those with strong will who desire to make the most of their abilities at a personal level (the people we call 'athletes'), and was contemptuous of those satisfied with their limited abilities. We may or may not agree, but so far the argument is harmless enough. The problem is that Nietzsche goes on say that those who pursue unlimited desire for power also evince an admirable strong will. Nietzsche allies this thought with a number of other unpleasant ideas, including his claim that the concept of human rights is just a ploy by those with weak will ('the herd') to protect themselves from those with strong will (the 'übermensch'). This disastrous philosophy gave sanction to Nazism.

Philosophers since Nietzsche (when they have not been advancing their careers and wasting their time 'proving' we have no free will) have been trying to get us out of this hole. They include Kafka with his stress on personal responsibility, and his warning that we are far too ready to surrender our free will as if to fate. They include Camus with his idea that we can always choose to fight against injustice, and they include Bergson who reaffirmed the justification for a belief in free will. It is some of this philosophical terrain that we have been exploring in the philosophy of dieting.

I should add that I have not in any sense been trying to trick the reader into reading a book of philosophy while pretending that it is a book about dieting. The book is about philosophy of course, but it also really is about identifying ways to diet that are practical and achievable and which promise long term results because they fit in more broadly with what you want out of life. My personal favourite is the bucket diet, perhaps because it fits with my liberal sensibilities and love of camping. All of the diets, however, even that of Nietzsche, are seriously meant. All provide genuine ways of losing weight.

Index

www.ingramcontent.com/pod-product-compliance
Lightning Source LLC
Chambersburg PA
CBHW060616290326
41930CB00051B/2656